RETHINKING HEALTH PROMOTION

A global approach

Théodore H. MacDonald

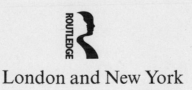
Routledge

London and New York

First published 1998
by Routledge
11 New Fetter Lane, London EC4P 4EE

Simultaneously published in the USA and Canada
by Routledge
29 West 35th Street, New York, NY 10001

© 1998 Théodore H. MacDonald
Typeset in Times by Routledge
Printed and bound in Great Britain by Redwood Books, Trowbridge, Wiltshire

British Library Cataloguing in Publication Data
A catalogue record for this book is available from the British Library

Library of Congress Cataloging in Publication Data
MacDonald, Théodore H. (Théodore Harney)
Rethinking health promotion: a global approach / Théodore H. MacDonald.
Includes bibliographical references and index.
1. Health promotion. 2. World health. I. Title.
RA427.8.M33   1998
613—dc21   97-41764

ISBN 0–415–16474–5 (hbk)
ISBN 0–415–16475–3 (pbk)

TO THE MEMORY OF
DAVID WIDGERY
PHYSICIAN AND SOCIALIST
AND
A MAN OF THE PEOPLE

CONTENTS

PREFACE

This text is intended to introduce the philosophy and content of health promotion to a variety of people. While primarily aimed at people who come from a health and/or medical (note that I differentiate!) background, the subject is of wide and increasing importance in the whole context of rapidly changing social and political values. Therefore, this offering is also intended to engage the thought and attention of a broad spectrum of socially-aware readers.

A number of attributes of health promotion immediately become clear even to a casual reader. For instance, health promotion is not the same thing as health education; medicine is an intrinsically *political* activity and not the 'neutral and dispassionate clinical science' that some are wont to think it is. Health promotion, if it is to define its scope of action rationally, must clearly delineate its relationship with clinical science and health education and this, apparently, cannot be done without some consideration of its social and political implications. But this, in turn, brings in issues related to ethics and philosophy. Indeed, it requires a fair degree of scholarly rigour to prevent a theory of health promotion from becoming that much sought after philosophers' stone, a 'Theory of Everything'! In a sense, of course, such a breadth is legitimate, for once we concern ourselves with problems of 'empowerment' and 'self-esteem', 'neighbourhood advocacy' and 'intersectorality', 'politics' and 'gender issues', etc., the whole gamut of the intellectual enterprise provides a legitimate avenue for enquiry. It would not be hard, for instance, to research a commentary on the link between Beethoven's *Requiem Mass* and the 'Concept of Autonomy'!

However, as I argue in this text, such an uncritically untrammelled approach does the study of health promotion no good. It makes of it a rather fuzzy repository of untested ideas and of anything which cannot definitely and decisively be encompassed by a clinical or medical model of some sort. Instead, the reality is that clinical science, like all science, is based on and advances largely on the basis of reductionist models. This is ideal for a narrowly defined problem – such as a specific illness. However, health is much more than freedom from specific illnesses. Its very breadth, as implied above, would render any reductionist model excessively restrictive. Yet that has to be the *vade-mecum* of clinical science and, accordingly, health promotion must define itself coherently enough for it not to simply include everything which cannot easily be medicalised.

To do this, I argue, we must delineate both the history and philosophy of health promotion's origins much more carefully than perhaps we have done in the past. Accordingly, in this book I include material on these topics in sufficient depth and rigour for the enquiring reader to properly appreciate health promotion's intellectual pedigree.

All of the topics addressed in this book are specifically addressed in the health promotion modules taught by this author in the MSc in Health Promotion at Brunel University College. In that respect, the material of each chapter has been trialed on students (approximately thirty in each cohort) every year since 1991. Over time much of the material has been modified, not only to keep it up to date, but in response to students' comments and observations.

No text of manageable size can address even all of the key issues in health promotion and, for this reason, I have had to exercise some degree of eclecticism in my choice of topics. For instance, environmental issues in health promotion are of enormous significance. Should I have produced a chapter on that? But, had I done so, word-limit constraints would have required me either to select some environmental issues while arbitrarily excluding equally crucial ones or to produce an inexcusably superficial account of the whole.

It will also be noticed that I have written with extensive and frequent use of references. This was done consciously and for two reasons. Firstly, health promotion could, as I have already indicated, become a grab-bag of unverified feelings and beliefs. The constant use of referencing, even for quite minor elements of analysis, serves to make this less likely. Secondly, students need to appreciate for themselves that their own good feelings and 'politically correct' assumptions are not a sufficient basis for analytical discourse unless they can be closely referenced. The intention is that, in such respects, this text be a model for them of good practice.

Health promotion, I contend, cannot really be called a 'discipline'. It draws parasitically on several existing disciplines. Nor would it want to be one if it is effectively to support the empowerment of individuals and of communities, for a 'discipline' presupposes a top–down model in which an authoritative body defines the issues and validates solutions. If health promotion ever becomes that tightly defined, then at best it will become health education only. Therefore, the reader will find that this book may answer some of his/her questions about health promotion, but it will (hopefully) raise far more questions than it answers!

For instance, health promotion (I will show) must have a 'global imperative'. However, the important features of its framework of enquiry are intrinsically eurocentric. How can we resolve that problem? It is hoped that the material discussed in this book will equip the reader at least to recognise that such questions are crucial to the enterprise and perhaps even equip him/her to begin to frame a coherent response

In closing this Preface, it would be most remiss of me not to acknowledge the many people without whose co-operation, encouragement and help this book could not have come into existence. Certainly paramount in this regard have been all of my health promotion students, both undergraduate and postgraduate, at Brunel University College from 1992 to 1997. Every chapter in this book has served as lecture material and each of the chapters has been refined over the past five years in the hot fires of student comment and criticism. As is ever the case with any academic writer, I must express my gratitude to my wife, Chris, and our son, Matthew, for the degree to which the authorship of this text has imposed on their constitutional rights over the past year. Their tolerance and forbearance in the face of the degree of neglect involved has been its own encouragement and it is appreciated. Finally, I must salute Andrea Boyes, whose patience in word-processing this entire document from my scrappy handwriting and from my even worse attempts at typing, has been truly heroic. May success long attend her own life as a teacher.

Théodore H. MacDonald
London
May, 1997

1

HEALTH PROMOTIONS ANCIENT AND MODERN AND THEIR RELATIONSHIP TO BIOMEDICINE

Introduction

In this chapter the author aims to show that the existence of 'health promotion', as an idea and as a framework for social policy, long ante-dates explicit use of the expression. It also sets out to make clear the epistemological differences between biomedicine (a largely reductionist exercise) and health promotion (an essentially holistic enterprise).

It has been rather well argued (Singer and Underwood 1962) that medicine in European civilisation has had two roughly parallel histories. The first was what we call the 'Hippocratic' tradition (although it started about 200 years before Hippocrates), which can be said to have run from about 600BC to AD200, 800 years or more. Then intervened a long period of religious persecution of scientific thought in Europe. We can hardly think of rational medicine beginning again in Europe until about AD1400. Thus our present scientific medicine has only had a lifetime of about 600 years, at the most. That is, it has not been running yet as long as Hippocratic medicine did.

The author argues that health promotion, likewise, has appeared twice on the stage, each time defined by the extent to which it has transcended the focus and the particularity which is the life-blood of rational scientific medicine. Space does not permit more than a sketchy reference to these developments, although the reader is encouraged to read Singer and Underwood (1962) to gain a fuller appreciation of the historical context.

Homer, in his *Iliad*, makes a number of references to the god Apollo as being the source of healing and of the knowledge of health. Since that was written *c.*1000BC, this Minoan belief was obviously well established by that time, although the Minoan civilisation itself was by then ancient history. According to the Minoan belief (Daremberg 1865), Chiron the centaur taught a *man* (not a god at that time) named Asklepios (and whose name goes under a wide variety of spellings) how to heal people and that was how humankind acquired the art of healing. Chiron gave Asklepios a staff with a serpent twined around it and in the various Asklepian temples which sprang up, once Asklepios had become a god, serpents played a crucial part in the healing rituals of the Minoans. Eventually, the story goes, Asklepios became so good at healing, that he could even raise the dead. Accordingly, Zeus struck him dead with a thunderbolt, as he was attracting too much adulation.

These particular details of the Minoan belief system seemed (in Homer's day) to have been confined to Thessaly, but a confusing element arises in the *Iliad*, for in that work Asklepios is still described as a man (a physician) while reference is made to two goddesses – Hygeia and Panacaea. But later sources (Farrington 1949) describe Hygeia and Panacaea as *daughters* of Asklepios. However, the relationship was differently perceived by different writers, with some later authors describing Hygeia as Asklepios' wife.

Dubos (1995), in his account of the gods of health, explains their different approaches to healing. Hygeia 'was the guardian of health who symbolised the belief that men could remain well if they lived according to reason'. The cult of Hygeia gave way to that of Asklepios who 'achieved fame not by teaching wisdom but by mastering the use of the knife and the knowledge of the curative virtues of plants'. As the popularity of Asklepios extended even beyond Greece, Hygeia became less important and was 'relegated to the role of a member of his retinue, usually as his daughter . . . but always subservient to him'. Panacaea, Hygeia's sister 'became omnipotent as a healing goddess through knowledge of drugs either from plants or from the earth'. Dubos suggests that her cult continues today as we seek a 'universal panacaea'.

Waldron (1978) suggests that Hygeia can be linked with the preventive or environmental aspect of medicine, whereas Panacaea specialised in the knowledge of drugs and represented the conviction that disease can be cured by the intervention of a physician. The latter represents the disease-orientated side of medicine. He comments that as medicine has developed through history, this division in approach has been preserved, with dominance afforded to intervention rather than prevention. Dubos suggests that 'myths of Hygeia and Asklepios symbolise the never ending oscillation between the two different points of view in medicine'.

Use of the gods in Rationalist Health Discourse

Hippocrates, whom Bellamy and Pfister (1992) suggest may have been more than one person, was pivotal in drawing our attention to a recognition of the links between a person's health status and his environment. They explain the ideas of Hippocrates in this way: 'illness is an interaction between the patient as a whole person, the disease, the healer and the environment surrounding them, and that the process of healing must invoke all of these'. They go on to refer to his belief in the healing powers of nature 'which the healer has to aid rather than replace, concentrating on the prognosis rather than the disease and using the diagnosis as a tool to this end'.

In another reference to Hippocrates the following has been written: 'his methods of diet and treatment prescribed have been said to be not unlike those of an intelligent if conservative general practitioner of about 1800' (Radice 1973). These ideas, it could be argued, indicate an enlightened attitude in demonstrating awareness of the influence of the environment on man's health when looked at from the perspective of the twentieth century.

Thus, by the time Hippocrates had written his Aphorisms, Prognostics and the entire Corpus Hippocraticum, it was perfectly evident that though he refers frequently to 'the gods' and especially to 'Panacaea and all the gods' (Larkey 1936) he does this as an atheist. This is especially evident in his Prognostics, in which he states categorically that 'the physician should not be guided by the words of oracles, seers and priests but only by what his senses are telling him' (Jones 1945). Thus his references to Apollo, Hygeia and Panacaea are convenient cultural figures of speech, rather that credal statements, in the same way that modern rationalists sometimes refer to feelings and values that at least temporarily are not accessible to the immediately empirical.

In that context, then, one recognises that often, when Hippocrates wishes to discuss such issues as self-confidence (*Hippocrates* 1926), community living, the role of music in healing, etc., he refers to the guidance of Hygeia, whereas in Prognostics, when he is discussing how to intervene, he 'swears by' Panacaea. That is, he held that Hygeia governed much of what we mean by 'health promotion', while Panacaea was regarded as the organising influence of 'medicalisation'. The fact that neither of these expressions existed until the 1970s cannot obviate the fact that the ideas they represent were there in Hippocrates' day and, moreover, bore roughly the same relationship to each other then as they do now.

The Hippocratic tradition's later years

It lies beyond the scope of this chapter to detail the growth and development of ancient rational medicine from 600BC to AD200. Suffice to say, Aristotle – who followed close on the heels of Hippocrates – was also unswervingly rationalist in his approach. His dissertations on logic, correct argument and ethics, along with his wide-ranging forays into descriptions of biological fieldwork, all reflect the same commitment to the evidence of the senses.

As Hellenisation took place in the early years of the Christian era, and just prior to it, the sort of rational medicine we have been describing flourished in the Alexandrian school, but in retrospect we can see that the seeds of its decline were set out in the context of its nurturing in the Roman Empire, for already there was developing, during those times, a tendency to adulate key figures and their writings, such as Aristotle, Plato, Hippocrates, etc. This was starting to have the effect of moving the focus of interest from observed illness phenomena to a semantic analysis of what could be deduced, by way of argument on the subject, from the writing of the 'great thinkers'.

Also, the Roman Empire represented a much more religious milieu than did the Greek, especially in terms of integrating religion officially into the life of the state. This author argues that both of these factors gradually killed off the necessary spirit of independent enquiry required to sustain rational medicine, or any other scientific enterprise for that matter.

The development of modern medicine

Although the interventionist approach has dominated medicine throughout history, Waldron (1978) reminds us that prevention has never been totally overlooked. He draws our attention to a medical book written around the thirteenth century entitled the *Regimen Sanitatis Salernitanum*, which laid down careful rules for the healthy life and cites the medical historian, Sigerist, who claimed 'there had never been a more successful medical book'. The book dealt with sleep and wakefulness, benefits of rest and exercise and with the qualities and effects of food and drink. The advice included the following:

> Rise early in the morne, and straight remember,
> With water cold to wash your hands and eyes,
> In gentle fashion retching eury member,
> And to refresh your braine when as you rise,
> In, heat in cold, in July and December.
> Both comb your head, and rub your teeth likewise:

> If you bled you haue, keep coole, if bath'keepe warme:
> If din'd, to stand or walke will do no harme
> Three things preserue the sight, Grasse, Glasse, & Fountains,
> At Eue'n springs, at morning visit mountains.
>
> (Waldron 1978)

This book, it could be argued, reflects the Hippocratic ideas and spirit.

Although rational medicine can be said to have had a new start with the Renaissance in the fifteenth century, after about thirteen centuries of torpor, it took some centuries to catch up again to where the ancient rational medicine had left off in AD 200, or thereabouts. Even a cursory study of the major outlines of that history, from, say, 1400 to the present day (Walker 1930), shows that it was characterised by bursts of optimistic activity around interventionist models whenever particular advances in medical knowledge were made. For example, Andreas Vesalius' daring and innovatory detailed anatomical work (on human corpses) encouraged a highly proactive and

4

heroically interventionist approach to medical observation, first among medical doctors in and around Padua but gradually, as the Italian Renaissance ideas took flight over the Alps, that attitude to the human body made its presence felt throughout western Europe and England. But between these 'major events', of which William Harvey's eventual discovery of how the blood gets from one side of the heart to the other is one outstanding example, medicine tended to be practised less optimistically and with greater recourse to 'received wisdom'. This was especially so with the use of strong mineral salts, compounds of antimony and mercury, etc. Many of these 'remedies' were derived by interpretation, often in a quasi religious sense, of 'venerable writings', including works by Aristotle, Hippocrates, Galen and others.

The focusing of biomedicine

As the tempo of medical breakthroughs increased (itself promoted by technological improvements in microscopy, etc.) the incidence of 'rational panacaeic' influences became more prominent. The influence of Hygeia did not diminish so much as to shift ground to areas less intensely medical and illness orientated.

Biomedicine's relationship with science must be explored if one is to make any sense of the argument that western Europe's emergence from the so-called 'dark-ages' was attendant upon a whole host of developments – the impact of Islamic culture through the crusades, the emergence of better means of exploration (e.g. the magnetic compass), the invention of printing, etc. We can truthfully say that the Renaissance and the rise of modern science went hand in hand. Pivotal to the development of the scientific approach is what we now call 'reductionism'. Put simply, science advances largely by focusing on as few variables as possible in the topic being investigated, ideally just two, so that one can be measured (a dependent variable) while the other (an independent variable) can be experimented with.

In philosophical debate one often hears the word 'reductionism' used in a pejorative sense, but in fact it is a technique of investigation which has largely underwritten modern science and all of the useful technologies derived therefrom. Of course, it is narrow in focus (reduced deliberately), but this renders it ideal for ascertaining the details of how things work. Once medicine applied reductionist thinking to illness, progress in the definition and eradication of disease served to separate biomedicine from health and to focus it on illness.

Health, of course, is much more than the absence of illness. It includes many variables relating to other people, self-esteem, economic status, etc. In other words 'health' is most certainly not an appropriate subject for reductionist techniques. Interpreting health requires an holistic approach, an approach that looks at how the variables interact without attempting to see some as 'independent' and some as 'dependent'. The interconnections are far too complex for that.

Thus we can say that since the Renaissance, biomedicine has focused increasingly on the productive use of reductionism in the study of disease, leaving 'health' to be investigated in a more open and holistic context. Reductionism is appropriate to the 'Panacaea' approach while holism lends itself best to what the ancients saw as that of Hygeia.

It must be realised, though, that even when medicine is here referred to as 'rational' and 'scientific' it was often neither. Old wives tales and/or hit or miss approaches, sometimes dignified with the sobriquet 'intuitive', were still the European physician's dominant stock in trade until the very late nineteenth century.

Bases of authority in modern medicine

This state of affairs ended abruptly and within a thirty year time span medicine became largely 'scientific' (governed by defined and accountable, objectively described natural laws) and, along with that, became much more narrowly focused on illness rather than on health. At least three general categories of development led to this:

1 anaesthetics;
2 means of securing accurate diagnoses;
3 insights into biochemistry.

When John Snow (Singer and Underwood 1962) anaesthetised women for obstetric reasons, using chloroform, he took a giant step in freeing medicine from the horrors of surgery done with no general anaesthetic. The book *The Reason Why* (Cecil Woodham-Smith 1991) graphically describes such surgery in the field hospitals at Scutari during the Crimean War. As far as pure surgical technique was concerned, the operations were often a 'success', but the patients usually died! – either of shock at the time or several days later due to uncontrolled infection.

The fact that anaesthetics (which rapidly evolved from the rather perilous chloroform stage) could allow surgery to be done reasonably safely immediately prompted much more daring forays into that field. Meanwhile, a more systematic insight into the chemistry of the sulfa drugs had, by the early twentieth century, reduced the likelihood of post-operative infection.

In fact, the sulfa drugs, and then later, about 1945, the discovery and availability of antibiotics, brought a whole new proactive attitude to play in the practice of medicine. In the art and drama of the time, the nineteenth-century doctor spent a lot of time dramatically hovering over his patient 'waiting for the crisis to pass'. His twentieth-century counterpart does not do that very often. Instead he/she administers an appropriate pharmaceutical.

Again, we do not have to go far back into the popular literature of the nineteenth century to realise that diagnosis was fairly hit or miss.

'Consumption' covered a multitude of conditions – not only tuberculosis. Symptoms were still often used to describe diagnoses – e.g. dyspepsia. The development of X-rays, stethoscopes, EKG, scanners of various types, histological preparation techniques, etc., in the twentieth century have all increased the precision of diagnosis immensely.

Thus, after about four centuries of sometimes being scientific, but more often not so, medicine now has a right to present itself as largely scientific and rational. However, while doing so, it has also suffered – to some degree – a loss of authority in the lay community. There are several reasons for this:

1   By becoming more precisely focused on illness-states, which themselves are more accurately diagnosed, medicine has largely marginalised itself from the mass of 'operationally healthy' people (Illich 1975).
2   The success of medicine has conferred on it extraordinary power which, in structural economic terms, ties in well with the capitalist corporate state (Navarro 1980). In this way it has alienated itself from large numbers of people, who now often tend to seek out friendlier and more accessible avenues of health advice.
3   It has been argued that top–down hierarchical authority structures, which medicine has assumed as a result of the highly specialised levels of education and technology it now embraces, are no longer perceived by many people as meeting their needs (Kassebaum and Baumann 1965).
4   Medicine has become marginalised further by specific attempts to 'deskill' it and to otherwise remove some of its power as part of a current tendency within some governments to delimit their level of responsibility for delivering healthcare. In the UK there is a growing tendency to accord recognition to, and to register, alternative therapies of various types. These are virtually all in the private sector and, if people can be encouraged to support them, it may lessen financial pressure on bodies such as the NHS.
5   It has been realised (McKeown 1979) that the development of medicine, as a rational discipline, had less to do with the health of society than had previously been assumed to be true.

With respect to the last item, not only was it realised that medicine had less to do with improvements in public health, but that political and social policy factors were largely to credit for those improvements. This realisation has empowered lay groups and individuals who find themselves outside of the austere hierarchy of the medical establishment. This author argues that this is one of the major thrusts behind the second appearance of health promotion.

Health promotion returns

As suggested previously in this chapter, health promotion did exist in conjunction with Hippocratic medicine, but not under that name. It made its appearance again – explicitly designated – in the work of Marc Lalonde (1974) and was soon incorporated in the Health for All initiatives of the WHO (World Health Organization). Ottawa was the venue of the first international conference on health promotion (November 1986) largely because Marc Lalonde was himself not only a Canadian, but was Minister of Health in that country when he produced the health promotion document referred to above.

Health promotion claims a distinct intellectual territory for itself in the following respects:

1   Any large-scale attempt to enhance people's health has to include many aspects which do not involve the biomedical orientation to the specific targeting of diseases.
2   Health education is certainly an important component of health promotion, but it is neither the same thing nor necessarily is it always in harmony with it. Health education involves the transmission of information relating to health. As such, it need not involve the people proactively.
3   Health promotion involves *empowerment*, a process whereby individual people are encouraged to assert their own autonomy and self-esteem sufficiently to be able to identify their own health agendas, rather than being told what to do or what is 'good for your health'.
4   Health promotion recognises that health is social as much as individual. Effective and healthy communities are sustained by 'neighbourhood advocacy' of various types – people identifying their health agendas as individuals and being sufficiently empowered to develop the necessary social and political skills to see how to tie it in with the neighbourhood or social health context.

Just as in its earlier development with Hippocratic medicine, modern health promotion is under Hygeia's influence, rather than Panacaea's and is likewise frustratingly subject to the interplay of religious and superstitious forces. Biomedicine, conversely, becomes more deterministic and empirical.

Conclusion

The general pattern, then, is quite clear. The history of European rational medicine has presented itself twice – the Hippocratic tradition (600BC to AD200) and the modern tradition (AD1500 to the present day). Each time it has attained authority through disentangling itself from the religious roots to which earlier generations had attributed its origins.

During the period of the Hippocratic tradition, the two goddesses who putatively guided physicians, were Hygeia and Panacaea, their human father (Asklepios) having somehow become deified in between. Initially, say from 1000BC to 600BC, these goddesses were widely accepted in that fully religious sense, with their favours being mediated by priests in appropriate temples. But the gradual emergence of the Hippocratic tradition, saw the gradual erosion of the temple's influence as the practice of medicine came under increasingly rational sway. The two deities, Hygeia and Panacaea, were still invoked, but increasingly as representing complementary attitudes to health, with Hygeia on the side of lifestyle and Panacaea on the side of biomedical intervention. Because the non-interventionist approaches, as reflected in the writings of the Hippocratic tradition, can be shown to parallel our current concerns with health promotion – namely 'empowerment', 'neighbourhood advocacy' and the eschewal of 'medicalisation' – the author has designated that entire development as 'ancient health promotion'.

Modern health promotion arose in much the same relationship to modern medicine as did ancient health promotion to Hippocratic medicine. Modern medicine also took some time to disentangle itself from religion and religious authority. As it did so, it became more specific and focused, leaving vast areas of health (as opposed to illness) to come under other forms of social construct. This, the author argues, was one of the principal thrusts to the development of modern health promotion. In parallel with the development of ancient health promotion, one can readily designate the Greek idea of a goddess Hygeia – as an attitude rather than playing a credal role in the development of modern medicine for the goddess Panacaea.

2

HEALTH PROMOTION: WHAT IS IT AND WHERE IS IT GOING?

In this chapter, it will be shown that once biomedicine and health promotion could be seen as best mediated by different approaches – reductionism for biomedicine and holism for health promotion – the role of ideology in both became more easily assessed. We shall consider the spread of the term 'health promotion' and show how it ties in with other ideas and movements in modern society.

One of the key phrases in health promotion is 'empowerment'. The author argues that the phrase is often used inappropriately because it has become a buzz-word, which is used to legitimise almost any health-related interaction between caregiver and client. It is suggested that one way out of the problem is to use different forms of the word for each of the two varieties of 'power-giving' – *impowerment* referring to power conferred on the patient or client by someone in authority and *empowerment* referring to the cultivation of a person's self-esteem to such a degree that they assume power over some aspect of their life, without reference to higher authority.

Empowerment is implied as a crucial element in both Lalonde's model of health promotion and that of WHOHFA (World Health Organization, Health for All) 2000, because health promotion is seen as engaging the community only after the individual has voluntarily interacted with his colleagues (neighbourhood advocacy) to promote an initiative which they perceive as important to their health. Such an element of trust in one's fellows would not normally be accessible to people of poor ego strength and low self-esteem. Only after neighbourhood advocacy has developed around an initiative can it be articulated (usually through political agencies) to involve the co-operation of such normally separate agencies as the police, government, schools, health authorities, etc. This is called intersectorality.

Origins and spread of the term 'health promotion'

The expression 'health promotion' has only been in existence (in the sense in which we currently use it) since 1973. At that time it appeared four times (in 60 pages) in a document *A New Perspective on the Health of Canadians*, personally written by the Canadian Minister of Health and Welfare, Marc Lalonde (Lalonde 1974; Bunton and MacDonald 1992). This document is significant because, not only is it extraordinarily rare for a minister to research and write his/her own publications in this way, but because it forcefully elaborated the point that all causes of ill-health could be attributed basically to non-medical origins! He identified four causes:

1   inadequacy in actual primary health care provision;
2   behavioural factors – both corporate and individual;
3   pollution of the environment;
4   bio-physical characteristics.

These were indeed uncharacteristically brave concepts for a government minister to advocate.

Moreover, it had its effect. The Canadian Government voted to change its then current policy away from treatment of illness to prevention of it. This appealed to the growing body of opinion, particularly feminist opinion (as shall be seen later in this publication), which had been articulating arguments against the 'medicalisation' of health (Basaglia 1986).

It was this initiative on the part of Lalonde which prompted the World Health Organization to mount the now famous Alma Ata Conference on Health Promotion, resulting in the *Alma Ata Declaration* of 1977 (WHO 1977). In the three years separating the two developments, the suitability of the phrase 'health promotion' as designating the multifaceted concept it does, had clearly become legitimated, for in the 120 pages of the *Alma Ata Declaration* we run across the phrase no less than seventy-one times.

Since then, health promotion has been the subject of books, papers and conferences uncountable, to the extent at which we could be forgiven for wondering how we even survived without it before!

What health promotion is and is not

Of course, the truth of the matter is that we have not survived without it any more than we have survived without attempts at medical care. It is just that throughout the long and tortuous history of the latter, health promotion has consistently been making its entries and exits to the stage, but well disguised and frequently anonymously. To appreciate this, we must now consider what health promotion actually is. Indeed, since it has so often been well hidden, let us accomplish this by reflecting on what it is *not*.

Health promotion is not the same as health education. Health education's brief is to acquaint people with the facts of what health is in explicit and identifiable terms, even empirically measurable terms. Teaching people how to look after their teeth and/or even how to draw a labelled diagram of the middle and inner ear, come under the ambit of health education. Likewise, information about nutrition is a major element of health education. Understandably, anything so connected with mortality as health education will have, over time, attracted a range of advocatory attitudes related to its preservation and mediation. Two such attitudes extant today are reflected in 'healthism', on the one hand, and in 'health promotion' on the other.

Healthism

Healthism uses health education as a repository of facts and information about body processes which can be made the subject of an individual's personal responsibility. The implication is that individuals are almost exclusively responsible for maintaining their own health through the exercise of informed choice. Thus, healthism emphasises personal decision-making about lifestyle and tends to see the body and its health as market commodities. 'You too can have a beautiful (desirable, healthy, chic, etc.) body' and 'happiness and health are both coterminous with success, wealth, significance, etc.' Healthism, so perceived, not only delineates these values as intrinsically and supremely worthwhile, it goes on to suggest that they are accessible through the simple exercise of wisdom and will-power: dieting, jogging, not smoking, etc. It also, by focusing on the attributes of personal choice and empirically measurable criteria ('how much weight have you lost this week?'), reduces access to a worthwhile life to the level at which delivery is channelled through the same market forces that determine, say, how many mono-grammed leather belts can be sold, where and to whom.

In the economy of healthist propaganda, people who so direct their slender resources have made a free choice and so can be blamed for their own ill-health. There are many aspects to this equation. For instance, how free is the choice made by those who have grown up as marginalised people in marginalised communities? To use one of the more dreadful acronyms bequeathed to our language by the Gulf War, and now enshrined in the 1992 Oxford English Dictionary, such people all too readily (and maybe accurately at that!) perceive themselves as PONSIs (People of No Strategic Importance). Do such people make 'free choices' or are their choices determined by the almost overwhelming need to be seen as participative in the 'real' society as conveyed by advertising, etc.? It is an interesting question.

At a more general level as well, healthism is often driven by 'victim blaming', in that people who accept the two basic propositions that:

1   the 'good life' depends on owning a 'body beautiful';
2   acquisition of a 'body beautiful' is a private matter involving personal choices about use of wealth, prioritisation of values, etc.

tend to see in the unfulfilled aspects of their lives a reflection of some dereliction on their part. Such derelictions are not hard to rationalise in this way, because most bodies manifestly fall short of the stereotyped 'body beautiful' image and this, in turn, can always be attributed to some sloppiness in the exercise routine or to falls from grace in the matter of following 'good' nutritional advice, etc. It rather forcefully reminds one of the Gospel dictum: 'He who would save his life shall lose it' (Matt. 16:25 NEB).

Healthism and the social context

While this preoccupation with sustaining a 'healthy body' can obviously lead to spiritual deprivation, somewhat less obviously, but no less surely, it can lead to social deprivation. For along with blaming the victim, it ineluctably encourages a philosophy that sees the wider society as, at best, irrelevant and as, at worst, an actual impediment. One must keep narrowing one's vision until one's own body (beautiful or otherwise) becomes the sole criterion by which values are vetted and strategic decisions made. It would be difficult indeed to think of a better way to impoverish social life and values (Rosenstock 1974).

Considerations such as the foregoing, then, make it evident that although healthism derives its material base from health education, it by no means embraces all of it. In an analogous way, as shall now be explained, we can see the relationship between health education and health promotion.

The term health 'promotion' implies an ongoing process involving both education *about* health as well as the elaboration of strategies which will enhance the effect of such education. It is this strategic aspect that informs us that health promotion involves a collective response (it transcends the activities and decisions of the individual) and, largely for that reason, is likely to seek (and find) expression through political structures and channels.

Health promotion

Today's health promotion, it might be argued, is underpinned by three major ideological/political thrusts:[1]

1 feminism;
2 environmentalism;
3 anti-authoritarianism.

The author has deliberately expressed these as 'isms', for in the sense that current health promotion attitudes give expression to them, they more often than not manifest themselves as strongly and philosophically advocatory and ideological.

As we shall see later, the historical reasons for this are highly informative and suggestive of a level of long-term coherency to the whole enterprise that is not obvious if the various phenomena are considered separately. For the present, though, let us consider each of these as 'legs' of the 'tripod' on which health promotion is supported.

Feminism

One of the roots of feminism, in the broadest sense, is that the origin and sustaining thrust to life is, and always has been, motherhood. Moreover, not only is motherhood basic in that regard, but the primary expression of motherhood is not only the act of giving birth, but the whole process of nurturing and protecting the young after that. Out of this grows the need to enhance life by avoiding unnecessary physical conflict and to positively seek out means of collaborating harmoniously with both the environment and with other people.

Many modern expressions of feminism appear far removed from this idea, but that it is basic to feminism *per se* can hardly be denied (Sayers 1982). Health promotion is a natural outlet for this creative, life-affirming aspect of feminism. But another aspect of feminism occupies an equally dominant influence in health promotion, and that is the feminist concern with the phenomenon known as 'medicalisation'. As we shall see, when considering the historical roots of health promotion, the development over time of medical knowledge has never represented the totality of general advances in healthcare and awareness and, at times, has been antagonistic to it (Zola 1975). For that reason, the term 'medicalisation' is more often than not used in a pejorative sense in the context of health promotion, almost as an ideological swear-word! Feminism's involvement with medicalisation has also frequently been adverse, the latter often being seen as representing male control over female health issues (Oakley 1980). By affirming a woman's right to control over her own health, especially with respect to child-bearing (as well as to other issues), the feminist movement has found itself seriously at odds with many of the entrenched social (and fiscal and political) attitudes of orthodox medical practice (medicalisation) and, therefore, often by default aligned with health promotion. This also ties in with the environmental and anti-authoritarian thrusts to health promotion, as we shall now show.

It takes little imagination to see that the pivotal role of 'feminism' in health promotion can be – indeed must be – generalised to address all forms of adverse social discrimination, e.g. racism, ageism, etc. This will become more evident when we consider health promotion's role in addressing issues of autonomy, empowerment, neighbourhood advocacy and intersectorality.

Environmentalism

The realisation that the physical environment sustains and nourishes us, and that we have a symbiotic relationship with it, is by no means new. All of the great religions implicitly enshrine such a view in their various creation myths, but it has only been recently (in historical terms) that we have been able to empirically measure both our deleterious impact on the environment and the length of time that we have left to remedy the matter. It took a century of heavy emphasis on industrialisation before we could even estimate the levels of industrially derived toxic wastes in the seas and it took yet more time to arrive at estimates of how quickly the seas could or could not reverse this damage and/or successfully sustain current rates of population growth. Measurements of atmospheric pollution and of the atmosphere's capacity to recover from such assaults took even longer. Sampling is just that little bit more inaccessible and the chemistry and physics required are just that little bit more obscure. Ten years ago, very few people knew about the ozone layer or its functions. Now most primary-school children in the UK can give some account of it (Prescott 1991).

Whereas health education could, and does, preach the aphorism: '*mens sana in corpore sano*', health promotion now points out that all this is very well but that there is no possibility of sustaining '*corpore sano*' in '*atmosfere poluto*'. Of course, the individual's capacity to prevent pollution of the atmosphere (and other environmental catastrophes) is much more circumscribed than is his/her freedom of choice in matters of exercises or diet. Concern for the environment is relatively ineffective unless it involves whole communities (Turner 1990). Indeed, the depletion of the Brazilian rain forests has taught us that even the nation-state is a fairly ineffective entity, as far as environmental protection is concerned. What people do in Brazil in the line of ordinary, non-military business and commerce – nothing terribly aggressive or high profile – can affect the health outlook of children in England as ineluctably as if the two nations were at war.

This realisation of our utterly contingent relationship with the welfare of the planet as a whole has led to the popularisation of the scientifically dubious idea of 'Gaia'. The term 'Gaia' itself is simply the Greek word for our world (planet Earth, if one likes), but the current Gaia concept goes far beyond this. It sees the planet plus its enveloping atmosphere (including the holey ozone layer) as an organism in its own right, struggling to re-achieve a sort of homeostatic equilibrium in response to each assault made on the total interrelated environment. Most of these assaults, of course, are made by humans.

The Gaia concept in that extreme form has been avidly promoted by the 'New Age' culture and its general lack of scientific validity is not regarded by the New Age movement as a barrier, since the movement also regards orthodox science as largely invalid anyway (Gardner 1991), the charge being that it is 'deterministic' and/or 'materialistic'. Rather than necessarily describing the philosophical attributes of science, it must be understood that many New-Agers use these two terms as ideological swear-words in much the same way that some feminist propaganda uses the word 'medicalisation'. Health promotion does garner some very high-flown swear-words!

However, the important thing about the Gaia concept is that it has made many more people aware of the seriousness of our situation with respect to the environment and it does hold out as our only hope the recognition that we must assume collective responsibility for it if we are to overcome the sure peril facing us. In this, not only does the 'Gaia' idea provide an important thrust to health promotion, but it ties in with the nurturing-motherhood aspect of feminism. Gaia is our mother and our nurturer. Dare we kill her?

Anti-authoritarianism by any other name

The author referred to the third thrust as 'anti-authoritarianism', for it is argued that such were its true origins, but many pioneers in the health promotion movement see it as 'empowerment' (Tones 1992). An explanation is in order.

Possibly because of the lack of the technological means now available to it, the mass media (newspapers and radio, if we antedate television) in times past did not undermine popular belief in the essential 'sense of structure' of our various social systems to the same extent as is now common. That is, with some exceptions, the media pretty well reflected the values of the *status quo*. People (again, with some exceptions) believed in their 'place' in the scheme of things and few seriously questioned the legitimacy of existing authority structures. The law was widely regarded as almost sacrosanct, lip-service was paid by many and sundry to the inviolability of the marriage-bond and of the duty of parents to children and vice versa, etc. God was in his Heaven (not his/her in *those* days!) and all was well with the world. One could quote many examples of the sort of thing to which the author refers.

It is difficult to put a precise date on the change in popular attitudes to authority. Some have argued that it represents a continuation of the questioning spirit engendered in the Renaissance. Others see it as a product of the Risorgimento in Italy. In this author's view, the emergence of the possibility of widespread and indiscriminate nuclear destruction (since 1945) has greatly weakened popular confidence in authority. Whatever the cause, it has engendered an attitude that does not sit easily with the idea of the classical 'doctor–patient' relationship, with the doctor's role being that of the thinker and the patient's role being that of obedience.

People thus left to seek security and purpose in 'doing their own thing' tended, when they did seek meaning in social organisation, to form 'special interest' groups in which they could delineate their particular needs as 'rights'. This presupposed a number of political and philosophical propositions about the 'legitimacy' of such social structures themselves but, suffice to say, it happened. Thus we had a proliferation of 'gay rights', 'women's rights', 'rights of children', 'save the whale', etc., groupings. The one feature all of these groups shared – and this is crucial – is a sense that their needs had been marginalised. What they sought was legitimacy and *empowerment*. Thus it is argued that empowerment as the third thrust behind health promotion is really a derivative of anti-authoritarianism.

'Empowerment' deconstructed

As stated at the outset of this chapter, 'empowerment' is widely used to refer to two distinct phenomena:

1 Telling people what is good for them and then assessing the degree to which the information is acted upon in terms of the fidelity of their compliance. This is frequently seen in health education contexts.
2 Creating a situation in which either a community or an individual is encouraged to acknowledge their own self-esteem and the legitimacy of their own autonomy and, on that basis, to identify their own health agenda and to organise themselves to bring it to fruition. This often requires community action and the health promoter accordingly finds himself/herself advising on educational, political or legal aspects. It can be a basis for neighbourhood advocacy.

The present author has suggested that one way around this semantic difficulty is to use the word *impowerment* for the first of these phenomena and the word *empowerment* for the second (MacDonald 1994). The overriding difference is that *impowerment* involves an input from outside oneself. One can truly speak of *impowering* people by giving them health information, instruction, etc., which they can then use to their health advantage. But *empowerment* must derive from the individual or community itself and this can only happen if the person or people involved have a high enough sense of self-esteem to recognise the legitimacy of their aspirations. Empowerment can thus not be an input, although it might arise indirectly from input if other information or counselling has led to an enhancement of self-esteem.

Empowerment requires, among other things, advocacy. The wider society, might be seen as hostile to the perceived and carefully researched interests of any given group. Rather than common values being taken as the touchstone, the current view might be that the social arena is really a competitive testing ground on which advocacy groupings fight it out. This simplistic view also fits in well with the 'market forces culture'. However, more thoughtful observers of the 'rights' scene, including many of its protagonists, have recognised that no group's rights are possible without being integrated with all other such right's. Health promotion, by tying this in with the other two thrusts of feminism and environmentalism, has provided a holistic and meaningful context for this empowerment.

Holism

At the risk of appearing to digress, it must be said that no view of health promotion can even pretend to be complete without at least a passing reference to holism. The term, along with such derivatives as 'holistic approaches' and 'holistic medicine', is such a commonplace now that one suspects that its real ideological significance, along with its interdependence with health promotion, are lost. It is said (Engel 1989) that the word 'holism' was first used by Jan Smuts in 1926. In using it, he was referring to phenomena much more immediately contextual to the South African scene of the time.

However, the modern use of the word is rather different. It has both a highly particularised meaning and a more general one, thus making it eminently suitable for ideological use! In the particular sense, 'holistic' is posed as the alternative to 'allopathic' in referring to models of healthcare.

Allopathic approaches (which accord with the biomedical model) are perceived as dealing with specifics of given disease states: symptomology, pathology, aetiology, diagnosis and cure. They are best accommodated by a reductionist approach. By contrast, a holistic attitude refers to the 'whole person' as he/she presents during illness. It assumes that the illness in some way reflects an imbalance within the matrix of influences impinging on the person from within and without, and that all of that taken together make the person what he/she is. Obviously, this latter scenario speaks much more sympathetically to the broad perspective of health promotion than does the orthodox biomedical model. It also provides (if one does not commit the rank discourtesy of looking too closely in some cases!) a legitimisation of such 'alternative therapies' as naturopathy, homeopathy, etc.

The more general meaning of 'holism', as currently used, derives from the strictly health context but is extended to include the person as a part of 'Gaia'. At this level, the term is so general as to almost be connotative only, like some religious terminology. But it does (through environmentalism) tie it in again with health promotion, conferring on it the dubious blessing of some very peculiar groups indeed. As mentioned already, the Gaia concept (as promulgated by New Age ideology) is non-scientific. However, one of the insights derived from the philosophy of science (Shapere 1977) is that it is rational to keep on using a defective model, long after it is known to be defective, if the concept it embodies ties together a number of other partly understood concepts. The 'Bohr atom' is an excellent example of this.

The Gaia concept, and the holistic view of man in it, may well be a fiction, but it is a germinal and useful one and ties together all three thrusts behind health promotion in a way that no other concept does. Myths, as we surely know, are useful and necessary.

Above all, these three thrusts reinforce Lalonde's view that health promotion cannot be seen as achieving a satisfactory resolution in purely national terms. It can have no long-term impact unless it involves Gaia as a whole. However, the concept of world-wide health promotion, as reflected in the WHO's targets of Health for All 2000, embody certain logical and philosophical problems. These will be addressed in the next chapter.

Note

1   The reader should note that this classification is not intended to replace the more usually quoted four-fold taxonomy of ecology, holism, equity and social justice; but to provide an epistemological basis for them.

3

ORIGINS AND INTERPRETATIONS OF FIRST WORLD HEALTH PROMOTION

The context of British health promotion

As described in Chapter 2, the reader will appreciate that health promotion, as we know and use the term, is very much 'context sensitive'. This is not only because of its link with the psychology of individuals, but because it depends on a large number of social variables which themselves are not easily measured. This is one reason for the appeal of reductionist models – they create less ambiguity. Health promotion, being holistic rather than reductionist will be deeply influenced in the form it takes by the particular contextual factors prevailing in a given society. For instance, in Britain, there had been a long history of public health. Until recently, however, people had tended to believe that the steady and measurable improvement in British public health had been brought about almost exclusively by progress in scientific medicine. This is certainly a view that the 'biomedical establishment' believed and promoted and, of course, it reflected well on it.

Basaglia (1986) showed that the great and measurable improvements in health over the past century in Britain have not, contrary to what such a simplistic view might suggest, followed on as a result of improvements and breakthroughs in medical science. The situation is confused in the popular mind because in the last century both general health and medical science have developed enormously and side-by-side. It is therefore quite natural to attribute the former to the latter.

What is now clear, however, is that the social organisation of health (in the form of public health initiatives such as sewerage systems, industrial labour legislation, etc.), rather than refinement of purely medical insight and power, has undergirded this spectacular improvement in popular health. Back in the 1950s the author's professor of biochemistry used to thunder in indignation that more people knew about Napoleon Bonaparte than about Alexander Fleming, and 'which man, I ask you, affected the lives of more people?' he would pose rhetorically. Now, forty years later, the author asks classes about the three men: Bonaparte, Fleming and Joseph Bazalgette. The first two are invariably accorded almost equal recognition (although

20

Napoleon still admittedly has the edge) but poor old Bazalgette hardly gets a nod. It was he who planned and developed the sewerage systems of both Manchester and London and, we now know, thereby saved more lives and contributed more to general health improvement than the whole army of microbe hunters of the day!

The significance, then, of this foray into the realms of comparative social status and sewers, is that no account of health promotion, either of its origins or of its significance, can be complete without investigating its involvement with public health.

The role of public health in Britain

The complete history of public health is edifying in the extreme, but for the more restricted purpose of delineating the significance of health promotion, the following proposition is defended. In the past 200 years or so, the relationship between Hygeia and Panacaea in the UK has gone one full circle. At the time of the French Revolution, Hygeia was gaining ascendancy, this gradually changed over the next century until Panacaea was dominant and now, since 1945, Hygeia is again ascendant and is represented in what we now call health promotion.

Another smaller pattern of periodicity can be seen in the nature of medical triumphs from 1860 onward. The old public health, as shall be seen later in this argument, looked for its legitimacy in defending people's health from outside agencies – germs, toxins, etc. As medicine became more and more accurate in first identifying bacteria, working out their connection with various diseases and their distribution and then elaborating *selective* methods for killing them, the old public health could respond appropriately by digging sewers, organising immunisation drives and preaching disease prevention. By the 1960s we had won most of the these battles, but people, it seemed, had stopped becoming healthier – or at least improvement in health indices stopped paralleling either medical developments (however measured) and sophistication in preventive public health. We were no longer threatened with outside agents so much as by our own activities and/or the effect that these were having on the wider environment on which we ultimately depend.

The new public health

This required a new response and a 'new' public health has arisen to meet it. This is characterised by a concern with social factors. These include large and contentious political issues, such as: the role of the tobacco trade in distorting the agricultural priorities of the third world with subsequent impact on malnutrition levels; trade relationships between nations leading to the wholesale destruction (by burning) of rainforests in order to graze beef cattle for meat export with subsequent impact on land rights of indigenous people;

deterioration of the ozone layer, etc. But they also include more locally constrained 'neighbourhood' issues, such as the psychological impact of certain types of housing, safety in the workplace, provision of optimum transport with minimum stress, etc.

While such issues certainly transcend healthism and go far beyond what can be achieved by individuals acting autonomously, they do involve empowerment of individuals rather than the reverse. Initially it may be difficult to see how this might be so. There is only a certain degree to which an individual as such can be 'empowered' as distinct from other individuals also competing for significance and dignity. However, until recently, individuals tended to think of their group affiliations in terms either of rather large blocs (such as one's nation, state or town) or of groups promoting a particular set of beliefs (such as church membership, political parties or unions, etc.). Only with the re-emphasis (c.1945) of the individual, brought about by the decline in the social legitimacy of former authority structures, were people stimulated to seek self-actualisation (Maslow 1954) through identifying with groups of other people like themselves.

We are now talking about groups of people formed from the 'bottom–up', formed to empower people experiencing a particular need, e.g. gay groups, sickle-cell clubs, etc. This phenomenon is almost diametrically opposed to that in which lonely or marginalised people join an already existing organisation or club (say, a church or a reading circle) as a solution to their sense of isolation. The former is empowerment, the latter is not necessarily so.

Now to see how all of this ties in with the 'new' public health and with health promotion, we must briefly consider the history of public health in Britain.

The history of public health in Britain

If we go back to what is generally regarded as the beginning of the Industrial Revolution in the late eighteenth century (Hammond (1950) puts it at 1760), the then prevailing situation was one in which 'public health' as such did not exist. There was no systematic social organisation of water supply or waste removal on a large scale. A consequence of this was that those portions of the community with the least economic power tended to sicken and die at rates far higher than those experienced by their more well-off countrymen – a totally unsurprising consequence. But a parallel consequence was that the populations of the financially deprived were not, at that time, heavily concentrated in towns and cities, so that the scourges which so shortened their lives did not pose a conspicuous threat to anyone else.

Of course, the Industrial Revolution (together with the various Enclosure Acts) changed all of that. The poor, now a proletariat poor rather than an agricultural poor (but bacteria are not particular), were not only more visible but represented a real infection danger to whole urban populations.

Orthodox medicine of the day, for all of its ignorance about the biology of pathogens, had at least ascertained the role of contagion, a role that was already well known by the time of the second Bubonic Plague epidemic of 1660 in Britain (Zinssner 1952). It was this fear of the effect on urban well-being of contagion that was the motivation behind the establishment of public health, rather than compassionate concern for the potential primary victims (Chave 1986).

Records of early meetings, for instance, of the Manchester Board of Health (Green and Anderson 1986) reflect an awareness that personal exhortation to cleanliness as an adjunct to Godliness, or even local remediation measures, would not be sufficient to stave off disaster unless national action was enlisted. These views, naturally, were those of the more enlightened, and the same records quite clearly reflect the level of indifference and active hostility to such concerns. However, as we know, factory reforms and public health measures gradually developed their own momentum as meeting the long-term needs of the capitalists of the day.

Edwin Chadwick, often presented as a champion of the urban poor because of his huge influence in bringing public health measures to fruition (Chave 1986), would probably be surprised were he to know of this role assigned him by an ahistorically-minded posterity. He is on record as having argued to a group of Sheffield industrialists that: the workhouses should be financed in such a way as to make starving on the streets just that little bit more attractive than 'going on the parish'. Widely disliked by both the landowners and the new moneyed industrial classes, the reason that he was held in opprobrium lay in the mistaken belief that his concern was for the poor. But in reality he was determinedly persuading the wealthy that it was in their interest to keep the poor from becoming massive sources of infection.

Recognition of the community's responsibility

Be all that as it may, it does not alter the fact that these first ventures in public health tended not only to protect people from outside pathogenic agents, but firmly established the principle that health had to be a community, as well as an individual, responsibility. In a very real sense, this brought public health to prominence. All of the great names in public health were recruited well before 1855 and public health in Britain had reached its zenith by about 1839.

What followed is most instructive, as far as modern day health promotion is concerned, and the author argues that to ignore such history is perilous, for by gaining ascendancy and access to political action, the public health movement progressively strangled itself. The Public Health Act (1848) permitted appointment of local Medical Officers of Health, who, in turn, became politically compliant over time. It also, of course, involved the medical profession with public health, a connection which until then had not been formally institutionalised. The Medical Officers of Health (MOH), 'professionally sycophantic' (Hart 1988) as well as politically compliant, in a sense expedited the 'medicalisation' of public health. The various 'Poor Laws', with their Draconian punitive measures, reflected this to a fine degree. Lay philanthropic activity, prompted by the same sort of fears that a generation previously had spurred people like Chadwick to action, rose over the supine MOHs in a bid to fill the gap, but this was easily divided off from the national political scene and arose in different ways in different districts in response to different priorities of problems. It was not co-ordinated and, more often than not, promoted the ideologies of healthism as a way forward. The community, if not lost altogether from the equation, became vastly less important to it.

This process can be amply exemplified but the author would direct the reader to the work of Julian Hart (1988) for this level of background information. Suffice to illustrate the general tendency was the emasculated Public Health Act of 1882, so hedged in by political compromise and medical professional antagonism, that the marginalised poor targeted by it tended to get 'defined out of existence'. Provisions were actually built into the 1912 Education Act to make it illegal for teachers to nominate children for free meals on a 'perceived need' basis, something which they had been doing since 1904. Instead, eligibility for the nutritional supplements actually mentioned in the 1882 Act had to be mediated by a severe means test and a rigorous medical inspection. In many areas, the latter could not always be easily arranged. The outbreak of war in 1914 improved matters considerably in the sense that legislation was soon in place to provide for free meals in schools. Other than that, it can truly be said that reforms evolved late and against both Ministry of Health and the medical/political establishment.

Health promotion – a consequence and a solution

It is in the context of such history that this author resists any attempt to confer on the study of health promotion the status of a 'discipline' in its own right. May it never become expert-ridden!

And here the story of the origins and development of health promotion is almost complete, with the history of public health leading us once more away from Panacaea into the influence of Hygeia after the Second World War, and for all of the reasons already given. For the 'new' public health, like the old, recognises that the interests of health require that individuals are empowered by defining their own needs and by organising accordingly, and that both political entrapment and professional arrogance are to be avoided. It is these realisations, in part, that make it different from the 'old' public health; that lead it to look at man in context and as part of the context, rather than as an isolated nobility assailed by essentially 'foreign' forces. We are talking here about an attitudinal difference, but it is, in essence, the difference between healthism and health promotion.

What will future historians say, then, about health promotion in the industrialised world? Will they, perhaps, select the time interval 1970–2000 as broadly comparable with the historical patterns I have described over the period roughly from the French Revolution to the present day? The comparison is not all that bizarre. The Acheson Report (DHSS 1981) slams the door on public health medicine's link with broader social issues. Does the 'new' public health, driven by lay involvement, empowerment and international protection of the environment, all acting through health promotion, confer on us control over the pattern and allow us to achieve a balance of good in the sibling rivalry between Hygeia and Panacaea?

Health and health promotion

Lalonde (1974) formulated a functionalist view of health. Within this view the components of human behaviour, environment, lifestyle and healthcare organisation, presented a new and comprehensive perspective on health. The fragments are brought together into a unified whole which permits everyone to see the importance of all of the factors (Lalonde 1974). One of the unique aspects of Lalonde's health field concept was the recognition of lifestyle as a powerful determinant of health. Inherently, the power base was shifted to a wider base of control: the people themselves. Interestingly, Chalmers and Farrell (1983) noted that perception of controls is an important determinant of health outcomes and will influence health promotion activities. Within Lalonde's view, health was clearly recognised to be holistic yet also subjective, notwithstanding the combined responsibility of the individual as well as his/her control of the environment. The WHO's current definition has moved beyond the biological causes, and views health more holistically and in its social context.

> Health is the extent to which an individual or group is able, on the one hand to realise aspirations and safety needs; and, on the other hand, to change or cope with the environment. It is to be seen as a resource for everyday life and not merely the objective of living. It is a positive concept emphasising social and personal resources as well as physical capacities.
>
> (WHO 1986)

In 1974, as stated previously, *A New Perspective on the Health of Canadians* was authored by Marc Lalonde, Canada's Minister of Health. The Lalonde document introduced the health field concept, which included the components of human biology, environment, lifestyle and healthcare organisation. With each component equally weighted, the paper outlined the importance of the individual and society, on determining health status (Lalonde 1974). As Raeburn (1992) clearly suggests, the Lalonde report signalled the intention to move almost exclusive controlling power in the health field away from the medical profession and biomedicine on to a wider base. Although viewed as a signal for the future in that health was conceptually expanded, in reality the focus remained predominantly on the individual and biological determinants of health.

Health for All 2000: The Ottawa Charter

In 1977, Health for All by the year 2000 was adopted by the World Health Organization (WHO 1977). The concept of primary healthcare was advocated by the WHO at the Alma Ata Conference held in the USSR in 1978. Since primary healthcare programmes provide promotive, preventive, curative and rehabilitative services, primary healthcare has been viewed as an important delivery strategy for achieving 'health for all' (WHO 1978; Little 1992). Equity in distribution and accessibility of all programmes were identified as key concepts in primary healthcare. In 1986, the Canadian document entitled 'Achieving Health for All: A Framework for Health Promotion' was released by Jake Epp, the Minister of National Health and Welfare. This framework identified health promotion as a multifaceted intervention designed to respond to the national health challenges of reducing inequities, increasing prevention and enhancing coping. Epp offered broad-based strategies and mechanisms that, if achieved by Canadians, could improve health and quality of life. Health promotion was seen as an approach to healthcare (Epp 1986). Epp clearly introduced the idea that achieving healthful states was both a personal and societal responsibility. Epp's framework was an attempt to do away with the 'victim blaming' which resulted from the heavy focus on individual behaviour following Lalonde's health field concept.

In contrast, Epp clearly addressed the fact that some people have unequal opportunities for achieving healthful states and that health is often related to factors beyond the individual's control. Epp's framework, which was presented later in 1986 at the International Health Promotion Conference in Ottawa, became known as the Ottawa Charter. The framework has since been viewed as a working document for action to achieve 'health for all' by the year 2000 and beyond. The framework outlined three health challenges for Canadians: reducing inequities, increasing prevention and enhancing coping. These challenges were offered as a means for Canadians to achieve health and improve quality of life.

Until the Ottawa Charter, there had been little effort to seek a consensus on the definition of health promotion. This author accepts the definition in the Ottawa Charter of health promotion as being, 'the process of enabling people to increase control over and to improve health' (Epp 1986). One believes that this definition gives added scope and purpose to health promotion. However, it may be quietly ignored or forgotten by the bureaucrats and politicians who attempt to make and carry out health promotion policies in their countries.

Because this definition implies a real shift in power in health from bureaucracies to people, democratic administrations cannot reject it, but they can resist it through benign neglect. Although the Ottawa Charter definition does not contradict others that emphasise the components or methods of health promotion, it raises a number of questions. For example: Why do definitions of health promotion evoke such quibbling and controversy? Part of the answer to this question must come from the fact that health promotion is one of the first and few truly interdisciplinary enterprises (along with public health) in health that seems genuinely emancipated from the domination of medicine. While medicine has its part to play in health promotion, the latter does not take its primary impetus from medicine or the medical model. The field of health promotion has been targeted by professionals of many disciplines, all of which are keen to contribute something to health promotion. This author argues that health promotion can be defined in practical terms as the combination of educational, organisational, economic and environmental support for action conducive to health.

Pinning health promotion down

The term health promotion is difficult to define, nevertheless a solid theoretical foundation of this concept is required if a full understanding and involvement are to be achieved. The term, health promotion, has often been used interchangeably with disease prevention, health maintenance and health education. Brubaker (1983) argues that the term health promotion is not synonymous with disease prevention, maintenance, primary prevention or health education. It is a term that does not refer to a specific area of health care. Health promotion involves movement toward a positive state of health and wellbeing.

While it has been suggested that health promotion and disease prevention are complementary, it is important to note that the goal of health promotion has a broader focus. Health-promoting activities strive to increase one's state of health, whereas disease prevention strives to maintain a *status quo*. Methodological approaches to study and evaluate health promotion are less developed than are those for disease prevention. While disease prevention research focuses on specific disease processes, health promotion research itself addresses health. Clarke (1992) argued that health promotion research is based on positivism. Positivism is rooted in a belief that it is possible to observe, describe, quantify and explain the social world as if it were objectively real, external and immovable (Clarke 1992). Health promotion is concerned with people and their wellbeing from their perspective (Raeburn 1992).

In health promotion, health is viewed as a positive construct and involves people in a participatory capacity. As participants, people are to be given as much control as possible to achieve health or a higher state of wellness.

Health promotion is grounded in philosophies of individual and community control of health (Townsend 1992). The quest for health and wellness within the health promotion area, therefore, becomes a responsibility of the collective as well as of the individual. Both societal and individual perceptions of health and wellness and perceived health status must be assessed. Behavioural components play an important role in health promotion, but social, economic, and ecological contexts also influence the process. In that sense, one can agree with Lalonde, that health promotion be viewed as a moral responsibility.

At the environmental level health promotion is the development of an environment that is conducive to overall wellness (Duffy 1988). Here, change in the social structure or environment is implied as being an important goal of health promotion activities. Although personal control and choice are implicit within health promotion, the focus has been extended to include a global perspective. Health promotion is not apolitical, rather it is an explicitly, politically orientated activity. Certainly, this should not be disguised, leaving the consumer (or provider) wondering about hidden agendas. Governments decide agendas and simply it is the authorities that set the priorities (Parish and Root 1991). Government agencies tend to portray a utilitarian attitude to consumers of health, citing the most good for the greatest number as the impetus for changes that occur in healthcare. Nevertheless, the fully informed healthcare consumer will probably perceive more control over health and participate to a greater degree.

While information may not always lead to greater actual participation, it is a requisite for *perceived* control and participation. Further, health consumers and health providers may increasingly be expected to become political and social activists in order to gain control and influence the factors that affect people's health.

To reiterate, the responsibility for health is both societal and individual. Health promotion is multisectoral, requiring a broad and holistic conceptualisation of health and healthcare by consumers and providers. In a broader context, health also includes empowered health consumers and professionals and a new generation of health services (Simard 1992). All this points to the concepts of 'empowerment' itself and this should be addressed.

Health promotion and the new public health

The principles and content of modern health promotion thus, it can be argued, are identical to those of the new public health. The principal aim is to effect national and local policy change to create social and economic conditions that promote rather than damage health. Health is affected by poor housing or homelessness, unemployment and low-waged jobs that are boring, demeaning, and dangerous. Above all, people are trapped in health damaging circumstances by poverty and low income. Not only is poverty associated with an unhealthy lifestyle, but, even when differences in lifestyle are taken into account, research demonstrates that socio-economic deprivation in and of itself harms health (Whitehead 1982). The promotion of health must, therefore, be linked to the transformation of social structures, policies and conditions that create illness, disability and premature death. Such changes in social structures doubtless require a redistribution of power and wealth, a handover of control from the wealthy and powerful minority to the majority.

Health promotion is generally agreed to take in three main kinds of activity, which often overlap (Tannahill 1985):

1 health education – communication to educate both those in powerful positions and the community at large about positive health, for example health groups, campaigns and lobbies;
2 prevention of ill-health – measures to reduce the risk of disease, illness, disability or any other unwanted state of health, for example screening for breast problems;
3 health protection – which stems from the more traditional public health approach; legal, fiscal and political measures, regulations, policies or voluntary codes to prevent ill-health and/or enhance wellbeing, for example, car seat-belt law, tax on cigarettes and alcohol.

Health promotion must be based on a number of principles, to avoid the pitfall of conventional health education. These principles include: reducing stress in the individual, rather than increasing it, because of a perceived gap between health and actual lifestyle.

Incorporating community development and participation and strengthening community action have to involve empowering rather than merely exhorting people to take more control of and responsibility for their own health and wellbeing, rather than worrying about matters of relative unimportance, and encouraging participation and a sense of belonging for particulate groups, such as smokers or HIV-positive people. Above all, the new health promotion must avoid the fundamental flaw of the old health education. The latter was based on an individualistic approach which 'blamed the victim', making people feel guilty about 'wrong behaviour', as though poverty, bad housing and other social pressures were non-existent. 'Victim blaming' makes conventional health education both ineffective and inappropriate for many social groups. The new health promotion, on the contrary, starts from the fact that the main causes of ill-health are socially, culturally and economically constructed and, as with unemployment, are often outside the individual's control. More importantly, appropriately organised, social action by the people concerned can often bring such factors within their control to a greater degree. Such must be the aim and a proper expression of real empowerment.

The Black Report and more recent work (such as Office of Population

Censuses and Surveys: Townsend 1992; Whitehead 1982) have documented the enormous inequalities in health between social classes and between different regions of Britain. The WHO policy document Health for All by the year 2000 included the objective of a 25 per cent decrease in such inequalities by the year 2000. Although the British government was a signatory to the WHO policy, inequalities have significantly widened in Britain in the past few years. Strategies to combat them must be part of government policy and, for any real impact, the will of government is crucial. Collaborative work is needed for local action by groups of health authorities and voluntary and community groups to come together to initiate local activities and to pool resources. Money and staff must be carefully targeted at the regions, districts, neighbourhoods and groups that most need them. But local health promotion programmes can only skim the surface of deprivation. An effective strategy must involve the redistribution of wealth and power in society.

Health promotion and the NHS

Health promotion in the NHS remains a peripheral and low-status activity. It is only within the past few years that some District Health Authorities have even established their own service and units with only one or two staff, and minute non-pay budgets still exist. The total inadequacy of resources is stressed because a very small service cannot be expected to fulfil more than the basic traditional role of providing leaflets, posters, and videos to health visitors and a small proportion of other health workers, together with some support to schools. Without more resources, the long-term development work essential for a coherent health promotion programme surely cannot be expected to take deep root in the NHS. Some of the large services have taken a step forward from the new health promotion by focusing away from the individual and on to the community and the institution. For example, the food and smoking policies now implemented in a majority of District Health Authorities have to some extent tackled the wider environment, by increasing the nutritional value of institutional food or introducing no smoking areas. However, the adverse conditions such as poverty, bad housing, and unemployment, that are often associated with smoking and unhealthy eating, are often either not acknowledged, or are mentioned but are then ignored. Outside the local health promotion service, a variety of other services are delivered to individuals by health authorities with the purpose of preventing ill-health. These include: first, ante-natal services, which include a range of screening tests, checks and health advice aimed at ensuring the birth of a healthy baby; second, children's health surveillance involving both developmental screening and vaccination and immunisation to support the growth of healthy children; and third, screening for cervical cancer and breast cancer which allows detection at an early stage in their development, when curative treatment is possible.

To be effective and useful within the framework of the new public health, all these preventive medical services must be approached with sensitivity to the social and medical contexts in which services are delivered. Communication with, and responsiveness to, the emotional and information needs of the people receiving the service needs to be a priority concern. Close collaboration between the healthcare workers involved needs to be maintained. Setting targets for achievement, continuous monitoring, quality control and evaluation should be maintained. Primary care is increasingly recognised as a valuable setting for health promotion. It can be defined as the network of services provided by a team of health and other workers from a health centre or general practice base to a small identified local population. The decentralised base of primary care might well be developed to enable more wide-ranging health promotion through participation in a range of information, activity and neighbourhood health groups.

Family Health Services Authorities, created in 1990, have great potential for the new health promotion. They are not dominated by the management of acute and secondary care services and the practitioners they manage are more closely in touch with community needs. In 1990, the GP contract introduced health promotion into the GPs' term of service for the first time and the decision to remunerate GP's health promotion clinics represents a substantial injection of resources. However, the opportunity of integrating primary care into the wider network of the new health promotion has been completely missed, as the regulations allow only the provisions of individual health advice in tightly defined circumstances. The 1993 GP contracts have gone some way to remedying this. It will be quite a major challenge for the new Family Health Services Authority to pick up the cause of community-based health promotion and the reduction of inequalities in health.

Possible recommendations

To become health-promoting, the author suggests that many health authority strategies would have to be reshaped in two fundamental ways. Firstly, rather than paying lip-service to the importance of collaboration by seeking support after policies have been developed, plans might have to be negotiated from the beginning in equal partnership with local authorities and community groups and a genuinely jointly planned and resourced strategy produced. There is a neighbourhood empowerment issue implicit here. Secondly, plans should focus not only on such problems as the prevention of heart disease or of cancer, but on people in groups within their environments, particularly in the workplace or community. Money and staff should be carefully targeted on a geographical basis to the most deprived communities in a region or district.

As Lalonde implies, health education and promotion are required at national level to provide leadership, develop materials and initiatives, fund research, disseminate information, co-ordinate the work of other statutory and voluntary bodies, run national campaigns, and most important, to challenge the policies of the health and government departments.

The mass media needs to play a vital role in health promotion. The government and the NHS health promotion services, after all, buy or negotiate space in the national and local press, on radio and television, for advertisements and coverage as part of campaigns to promote healthier lifestyles. These media, therefore, remain a relatively powerful means of informing and promoting public discussion about the impact of social, economic and environmental issues on health, of tackling inequalities and of fostering community participation.

4

HEALTH PROMOTION: A
EUROCENTRIC PHENOMENON

The paradox

As we have seen, health promotion can only make sense as a 'global' phenomenon. It would be no use for Canada, say, to have a 'national' health promotion policy which did not take account of environmental factors imposed on it by, say, Mexican or American activities that affect atmospheric pollution in Canada. While this sort of thing is readily enough acknowledged, the difficulties attendant upon circumventing it have not attracted a great deal of analysis. The fact of the matter is that what we, in the industrialised, 'European' cultures, refer to as 'health promotion' is by no means a culture-free entity. It is solidly based, for instance, on the concept of 'individual autonomy' and that is by no means a universal outlook on the condition of humankind. In fact, as with a great many of our cultural values, we can easily trace the concern with the 'individual' in history, society and politics, to the ancient Greeks. It is a phenomenon which does not apply with the same force in non-European cultures.

There are alternatives to the Graeco-Roman view of man. In many societies, the 'collective', be it one sort or another, is of immensely more significance than is the individual person. If one goes to, say, Nepal, with the idea of promoting primary healthcare, one quickly realises that models which work well in Europe or in the US make huge assumptions about the primacy of the individual's importance and cannot be directly applied in a situation in which the extended family or the tribe are paramount. Yet about two-thirds of the world's population belong to what we call the 'third world'. If health promotion really is to assume global applicability, there are a number of factors we must consider. Among these are: Do 'empowerment' and 'autonomy' have parallels in the social psychology of cultures in which individualism is not regarded as a primary virtue? How is western psychology different because of the importance of the individual to us? To what extent are societies fixed in their attitudes toward such issues as individualism and collectivism by their origins and backgrounds?

33

European individualism

It goes without saying that many of our western values and traditions are rooted in Greek thought. Because of this, many people tend to think of the ancient Greeks as being intrinsically 'wise' and/or 'profound'. However, one does not have to read much of Greek literature to recognise that in many ways they were surprisingly restricted in their view of humanity. For instance, they were terrified of deformity of any kind. Stories such as *Theseus*, *Oedipus Rex*, etc. make it quite clear that the ideal person was free of 'blemish' (tall, lithe, good-looking, fearless, etc.). Men were of much greater importance than women, physical appearance was crucially important and, above all, the figure of 'the hero' (a Greek word itself) was paramount. The 'hero' was never *part* of society, and certainly not *representative* of it. He (usually male) reflected a contempt for many social expectations and norms, while at the same time being rapidly and intolerantly conformist to others. His distinguishing attributes marked him as opposing natural forces, regarding such phenomena as somehow hostile and to be overcome by courage and perseverance, rather than factors with which to be acquiesced. The Greek hero, typically, was not a 'social being' but stood alone and defiant. Aggression and combativeness were his hallmarks while, by implication, co-operation with one's fellows and acquiescence and flexibility in the face of natural forces were regarded as weaknesses. As stated earlier, deformity was definitely looked down upon and, in much of Greek literature, was taken as a sign of divine disapproval and a curse. For instance, in the play *Oedipus Rex*, by Sophocles (1924), the crucial thing about his swollen foot was that, even though he was 'straight and tall, courageous and waxed strong in the eyes of man and the gods', the audience knew that his deformity as a baby marked him out ultimately for a degrading fate.

Now this may all sound terribly remote and theoretical, but it is of immense importance to us as 'Europeans' because those attitudes inform all of the rest of our philosophical religious and social values. We have superseded them only by conscious will, by counterposing other more morally acceptable models, but even these retain the dominance of the individual as opposed to society. For instance, the Judaeo-Christian view of man at first glance is in many ways different from the 'hero' view because it emphasises love, forgiveness, compassion for those broken in body and spirit, etc. But its theology could easily be 'fitted in' with ancient Greek values, especially through the work of the Church Fathers such as Thomas Aquinas, through his analysis of the writings of Aristotle.

Historically and culturally this has given us a mixed message and a mixed model down through the ages. It was but a short step from the view of life that all people are in some way important as individuals to the view that individuals have no meaning apart from society as such. Various socialist ideologies, of which Marxism has certainly been the most prominent, have given expression to this view. Clearly, in societies run along Marxist lines, empowerment of individuals (and the attendant preoccupation with autonomy and self-esteem) takes second place to neighbourhood advocacy, which in turn must presuppose intersectorality of government bureaucracies. Thus, even within the 'European' tradition, the protocols which gave rise to what Lalonde (and later the Alma Ata Conference) called 'health promotion' do not appear to apply universally.

This author (MacDonald 1996) has pointed out that in Cuba we have possibly the most successful example of health promotion and yet structurally it reverses in many respects the order and sequence of social-psychological forces which we, in the European mainstream, regard as canonical. It goes without saying, therefore, that once we move outside of the European tradition altogether, something which we must do if we are to consider health promotion in the third world, the differences will be even more marked.

Impact of imperialism on culture and consciousness

However, attempts to carry out any analysis of these differences and their implications are rendered much more difficult by the dependency relations, in terms of international trade, between third-world societies and our own. Indeed, and more subtly, these factors of what might be called 'economic imperialism' are deeply underwritten and sustained by a pervasive 'cultural imperialism'. To give an example, we in the European tradition have defined the academic discipline of 'psychology'. For the sake of argument, we can base its emergence as a separate discipline on the work of Sigmund Freud, a devout apostle of the Greek 'hero' approach.

But precisely where we start hardly matters. The point is that we in health promotion must be conscious of the fact that there are two 'psychologies'. There are those emotional and behavioural phenomena which differ from society to society and which are designated as 'psychology', of the sort which we have defined. Our relative economic power has insured that when, say, a Papuan talks about psychology as a discipline, he is speaking of it in our terms. But to what degree is he even aware of the fact that such academic psychology may not be describing the reality of his own ethnic psychology?

This crucial issue was dealt with in 1993 by the British Psychological Society in a series of papers in its journal, *The Psychologist*, and we shall be considering some of this material later in this chapter. Suffice to say that, if we wish to delve into the provenance of empowerment, psychology is the discipline on which we must focus our attention. Whatever one may think about Sigmund Freud and his system of psychoanalysis, his influence on peoples' insight into matters psychological has been pivotal in the development of western psychological models.

The Freudian view of humankind

Before describing the Freudian model as such, the reader should appreciate the comparatively narrow base on which it was derived and its social class origins. Freud developed his theories in late nineteenth-century Vienna on the basis of consultational experience confined almost totally to upper-middle-class Viennese women. In the brief summary of his ideas which follows, the author will only focus on those aspects which relate directly to the psychodynamics of self-concept, autonomy and hence of empowerment as thought of in the health promotion context. Nothing will be said about such hugely important aspects of his work as the possible origins of his views on women's sexuality or other controversial issues. If the reader is not already familiar with this material, this author would urge a hasty remediation of the deficit. There are many good and accessible positive accounts of Freudianism (Freud 1953), and a commendably thorough negative view has been given by Masson (1992).

All existing psychodynamic models, those of Jung, Erikson, Klein, etc., even though they each oppose Freud in crucial details, incorporate large parts of his model. This author would argue, therefore, that a clear insight into empowerment is not possible without a knowledge of the Freudian model.

Freud was of the opinion that personality development is strongly linked to what he called the 'libido' or 'sex drive' and that this develops in all individuals in a roughly similar succession of stages. As he saw it, most psychological illness stems from disturbances or dysfunctionality in one or more of these libidinal stages. With such a model, it is obvious that a child's psychological development will be strongly influenced by his/her parents and by other intimate prestige figures. One of his most well-known accounts of this is embodied in his book *Beyond the Pleasure Principle*, in which he declared there to be two basic drives which mediate personality. These are the Eros (love) drive powered by libido (sexual) energy. This, though, is balanced by the Thanatos (death) drive which derives from a death-wish and is often expressed in aggressive behaviour (Freud 1984a, 1984b).

To explain how all of this holds together, Freud postulated that the mind consists of a 'region' of cognitive awareness (called the 'conscious'), which includes all of those issues and events which are accessible to voluntary use by the person at any time, and of a much larger and growing 'region', which includes time, issues and events which once were part of our conscious experience but have since been stored away, sealed in, so to speak, by a 'repression barrier' in what he called the 'unconscious'. Material from the unconscious only crosses into the conscious in dribs and drabs and under special circumstances, as during dreams. Psychoanalysis involves helping a patient become conscious of certain material buried in the unconscious with the intention of the patient gaining insight (and hopefully control) over destructive psychological states of which he/she is victim.

Ordinarily, though, the purpose of the unconscious is to allow the person to reach an optimum relationship with society and thus to be as effective as possible. Therefore, much of the material buried in the unconscious consists of memories of events which do not fit in with a view, on the part of a child, that he/she can trust the powerful adults around him/her and on whom he/she utterly depends. Freud hypothesised that, unless such a mechanism existed, the person's sense of wellbeing (and hence their potential for empowerment) would constantly be threatened, but to understand this claim it is necessary to give a brief account of his topographic tripartite structure of the mind.

The topographic structure of the mind

Freud's idea of the mind being 'administered' by the id, ego and superego has never been substantially rejected, even by those psychodynamicists who subsequently have been most hostile to his view in other respects.

The id is a basic mind structure, fully operational at birth, with a drive directed toward gratification of the baby's needs and feelings and without any regard to other constraints. In Freud's view, the id operates without regard to 'external reality', it is entirely without any sense of time, for instance. It is not affected by logic or reason and is concerned with the baby's needs and instincts, such as its biological needs for food, warmth and its emotional needs for libidinal gratification. The id is prompted by impulses which produce tension and that require neutralising by being satisfied. Once the tension has been released the person feels a decrease in frustration. In this respect the id represents the infantile personality and is directed only at the survival of the weak and small baby, utterly dependent on the goodwill of adults stronger and larger than itself.

Further development requires the ego. Once the child starts to become independently mobile and able to use speech, even at a rudimentary level, it can begin to exercise some autonomy. But this requires that it be guided by a mind aware of 'reality', of time constraints, consequences, cause and effect, etc. This is the job of the ego. It is still directed at mediating the gratification of needs, but in such a way as to minimise the possibility of conflict with other ego-driven individuals. That is, the ego recognises a social dimension. The ego, being governed by the 'reality principle', can distinguish between wishful thinking and fact. It is able to defer its need for gratification by taking into account the consequences of the act on other peoples' reactions. Thus, in the Freudian view, the person's mind is mediated by the id and the ego by about the age of 30–36 months. The id operates entirely at the unconscious level, but the ego operates at both conscious and unconscious levels, as follows.

The conscious part of the ego, that part which controls the cognitive processes by which the developing person makes decisions which affect his/her very survival, must be protected from serious ambiguities that could render it unable to operate cognitively. Thus, if the ego encounters events which compromise its integrity or survival and if an event is of such magnitude as to render it impossible for it to be accommodated by the mind's developing cognitive framework, it will be pushed 'below' the repression barrier into the unconscious. For instance, a child's survival requires that it implicitly trusts the more powerful adults who care for it. Suppose one of these were to sexually abuse the child in his/her care. The child could learn thereby to reject that adult, but this would compromise its cognitive pattern on which it relies for coming to daily grips with reality. Therefore, instead, such episodes are repressed. The child, of course, knows that they have happened but, at the time, it is more cognitively consistent for him or her to accept these events in the terms presented by the abusing adult. That is, usually the young child assumes guilt for the pain and loss he/she feels and, although this will certainly depress his later ego development and sense of self-esteem, it does allow him/her to survive. Later, perhaps in adulthood, crippled psychologically by a sense of low self-esteem, the person may consult a psychoanalyst who, through regression therapy, will confront the patient with what really happened and, with this insight, the person might regain the capacity for empowerment. The reader will appreciate, of course, that this has to be stated in very simplistic terms in such a brief overview.

It is the 'defence mechanisms' defined by Freud, which provide the means for suppressing material and memory of events which threaten the integrity of the ego. These defence mechanisms include such well-known ones as rationalisation, interjection, sublimation, identification with the aggressor, etc., and the reader who is unfamiliar with these would do well to study the phenomenon in great depth in order to really understand the significance of self-esteem, autonomy and empowerment in health promotion (Freud 1991a, 1991b).

In the Freudian model, it is not until the person is six or seven years of age that the superego enters the scene, as a result of the child resolving the well-known 'Oedipal complex'. The superego is, for want of a better turn of phrase, the 'voice of social control'. It can be thought of as the person's 'conscience' in the sense that it acts as a censor over the person's thoughts, alerting the person to what is 'right' and 'wrong'. Of course, these terms have no universal application across ethnic cultural lines in the sense that an action or thought approved of by a British superego might well be disapproved of by a Solomon Islander's superego. The important thing is that the superego exerts guidance over the ego, inducing it to conform to the norms of a particular society. Freud thought of it as itself being subdivided into two parts as follows. The first part (or 'censor') is within the conscious mind and threatens the ego with punishment (in the form of guilt, usually) if it prompts thoughts or entertains impulses which are not socially acceptable. The second part is buried in the unconscious and rewards acceptable processes in the ego with a sense of heightened self-esteem. To a greater or lesser degree, the integrity of the ego relies on it being able to manoeuvre so as to maximise positive input from the superego and to minimise negative input therefrom.

The Freudian account of self-concept

It can now be explained how this model is so pivotal in accounting for the individual's self-confidence and how this is basic to the processes which underlie empowerment. All of this is dependent on the self-concept and is entirely consistent with the view that the individual, in a sense, transcends his/her society (a perfect reflection of ancient Greek values and still leading a robust life in the industrialised societies!). Freud defined as 'self-concept' all the thoughts and feelings which relate to how an individual perceives his/her own personality. This capacity to perceive oneself, as though somehow being an external observer, requires a sense of moral judgement and this cannot be mediated until the superego is in place.

According to Freud (1991b), and as implied earlier, the superego comes into operation once the oedipal complex is resolved. Freud gave it that name after the famous tragedy by Sophocles in which Oedipus, a foundling baby, is raised by a couple whom Oedipus does not know are not his real parents. He unknowingly kills his real father and then, also unknowingly, marries his real mother. Freud used this well-known classical tragedy to describe the incestuous feelings a young boy has for his mother ('when I grow up, I'm going to marry Mummy') and the attendant jealous resentment he has toward his father, who seems to occupy so much of his mother's affection.

Eventually the boy accepts that his father really is more powerful than himself and he starts to remould his behaviour on the fear that the father might divine his antagonism and punish him by cutting his penis off, a fear which, rather inaccurately, Freud called the 'castration fear'. The boy accordingly tries to conceal his 'intellectual treachery' by taking on many of his father's mannerisms in the hope that his father will look on him compassionately. This, of course, is one of the 'defence mechanisms' (identification with the aggressor) mentioned earlier. As this happens, he incorporates his father's authority into his own mental apparatus so that, in a sense, he becomes submissive to his father's will. This is none other than the installation of the superego.

Girls undergo a similar superego development. Freud suggests that, between the ages of four and six years, the girl envies her father's penis and blames her lack of one on the feeling that her mother 'castrated' (Freud's term) her. She therefore transfers her affection to her father but eventually becomes more ambivalent about the matter as the realisation sinks in that she cannot replace her mother. The effectiveness with which each individual copes with the resolution of the oedipal complex, within the context of western psychodynamic accounts, determines how robust a person's self-esteem is and therefore their capacity for empowerment.

Empowerment as a eurocentric phenomenon

But what of ethnic systems which do not derive their cultural values from such an individualistic focus? The fact is that, when people from third-world societies study psychology, they study it as an international discipline and are, to a large degree, unaware of the extent to which it is eurocentric and may not be describing 'psychology' as it is experienced in their culture. The belief that what they are studying is neutral tends to obscure these important differences. However, such differences do not go out of existence on that ground and there is no particular reason for assuming that what works for health promotion here may not work for health promotion in a third-world society.

In 1969, John Berry postulated a basis for analysing the behaviour patterns of different societies. To do this, he derived much from the work of Pike (1966) who had investigated phonetics (general analysis of speech sounds) and phonemics (analysis of speech sounds in *one given language*). Pike had suggested two complementary types of analysis and he called them *etic* (generalised culturally independent features) and *emic* (referring to studies within one culture). Berry applied this idea to the study of psychology of different cultures.

Riger (1993) supports Berry in his contention that a western cultural perspective has been imposed on all of the world's cultures. Berry suggests that the way forward is to establish which behaviours in any two different cultures are functionally equivalent. From these behaviours categories and concepts can be identified and then used to form an etic which can then be imposed. This newly imposed etic can then be modified by the people concerned, but without losing the main attributes of the culture. This constitutes a *derived emic*. The derived emic can, through group discussion, become a *derived etic*. If this could be done, it would address the problem of rendering health promotion 'global' because it would maintain 'autonomy development', but not at the loss of cultural reference points.

Another important contributor to this important debate has been Airhihenbuwa (1993, 1994) who asserts that the concept of empowerment, as we use it in health promotion, is heavily eurocentric. The author raised the issue (MacDonald 1996) in another context with reference to societies adopting a Marxist approach to social policy. Airhihenbuwa argues that western health promotion models trivialise the effect of cultural diversity within many African societies by placing so much emphasis on western models of learning and discourse based on the written word. As has been argued by this author (MacDonald 1983), the western preoccupation with print, based on the assumption of widespread literacy, imposes its own approach to linear thinking and sequencing. These do not apply in a society in which information is spread laterally, through communal intercourse, rather than from books distributed by an authoritative repository of knowledge.

As Airhihenbuwa describes it, our eurocentric model of classical pedagogy has disempowered African children when it comes to health promotion. He argues that health promotion in the third world should base itself on empowerment of communities, rather than of individuals, and he gives a number of examples of how health promotion has been mishandled in Africa through attempts to mediate it along western lines.

Psychology as cultural imperialism

But such advice ignores the political and economic realities imposed by the unequal trading relations between the third world and the first. The author has already referred to the debate on this problem which livened several issues of the *Bulletin of the British Psychological Society* in 1993. We now return to those contributions.

Basically the problem is this. If a bright student in a third-world society can gather the resources and study psychology at one of his country's universities, he will learn it from western textbooks. Indeed, until recently, he/she would have been likely to take degree examinations from the University of London and compete for his/her qualification on a 'level playing field' with students from other countries, including Britain. The papers would have been graded by British professors using western psychology as the yardstick against which all of the student's responses would have been graded. But that is not all. If our hypothetical student is very talented, he may be given the opportunity to do postgraduate study in psychology in one of the more prestigious western universities. On completing his/her doctorate, he may see a senior position in Psychology advertised in one of his/her own country's universities and apply. He/she would almost certainly secure the post and thus convey to prospective students of his own ethnic group even greater credibility as representing what 'psychology' is. But, of course, he/she knows no more about the psychology of that culture than did his European mentors, for he has become an expert in western psychology.

The real question is: To what extent does this kind of 'casual' cultural imperialism translate to hard-nosed explorative imperialism? Letlake-Rennery (1993) argues that it does. Writing at the time just before the apartheid regime had collapsed in South Africa, she made the following comment:

> South African psychology is about the great denial. Presently, White psychologists deny the existence of differences among people. They feel that if they do acknowledge these difference it will show how inadequate they have been in facing the problems of the majority of the South African population. This is difficult for White South African psychologists to hear, so it means that the situation at the moment is polarized. Because of historical reasons, all the resources, power and decision-making capacities are in White hands and at present there is no sign of a unified front against oppression.

It is very safe for me to say that the only reasons progressive White psychologists are willing to have contact with Black psychologists is to access resources and avenues that will enable them to continue the *status quo*. In other words, it has become fashionable to research Black populations and question racism and oppression, but only as far as to enable progressive White psychologists to go overseas and internationally represent South Africa and themselves.

. . . American psychologists engaging in professional support for South African colleagues should be aware of what their colleagues do rather than what they say. Are psychologists of color achieving positions of responsibility, or are they just employed as tokens for an image of integration? Is research conducted to empower and engage the majority of the population or is it conducted as a means of disenfranchising the quiet masses?

Is psychotherapy concentrating on the cultural and socio-political diversity of a country after 300 years of oppression, or is it the attempt to cement eurocentric categories as models for the explanation of psychological problems?

(Letlake-Rennery 1993)

The author presents that comment in full because it so poignantly addresses the issue and makes it abundantly clear that one cannot regard psychology as a 'neutral science' to be applied world-wide. In the next issue of the Bulletin, Stephen Davies of the Institute of Psychiatry in London comments on the dangers of making that very assumption. Not only psychology, but all of the health sciences, are able to very effectively deny a peoples' cultural integrity by playing the 'neutral science' card, even to the extent that those attitudes contributed effectively to the maintenance of the apartheid state. No person can be 'empowered' if the intellectual tools they are given with which to work and to validate their empowerment in fact deny the legitimacy of their own communal experiences. He even goes on to argue that:

This is true of South African clinical psychology but also of the profession in Western countries. Black people have generally been poorly served by mental health services which must mean psychologists as well. We white psychologists still need to remind ourselves that this fact cannot make the profession all that attractive for black people to enter or to use.

(Davies 1993)

All of this raises terribly serious issues about the importance of community validation of what may, on the surface, appear as scientifically neutral psychology. Among psychologists themselves, who may not be aware of the wider health promotion implications, there will be some who are quite prepared to apply their discipline to individuals in third-world countries in the spirit of neutrality described above (Reeler 1991; Tembo 1991; Foster and Louw-Potgieter 1991), while others declare that the cultural conditions and the distortion imposed on these conditions by disadvantageous trading relations with industrialised nations render it impossible to use traditional 'psychological science' in the third world in the way in which it is used in the first (Akin-Ojundeji 1991; Antaki 1989; Harris 1990; Jahoda 1983; Omari 1983; Smith 1991/2; Sinha 1983).

What all of this suggests is that we face a serious anomaly in health promotion. Its full value, impact and use cannot be appreciated by applying it within one country or society (Lalonde 1974). Its imperative is a global application. But our psychological insights into the necessary preconditions for the development of empowerment, on which health promotion is based, are so strongly eurocentric as to possibly render them invalid if applied outside of that first-world context. Unless and until that problem is addressed and resolved, health promotion will languish on the vine as a compelling intellectual and social argument with no means of being applied.

The future of third-world health promotion

Much of the foregoing might have struck the reader as somewhat irrelevant, but hopefully what follows will show that such is far from the case. What has been argued so far is that health promotion, as it has developed in the industrialised west, is a product of European psychological values and insights. In other words it is 'eurocentric' and thus cannot be regarded as a neutral product of scientific thought that can be applied readily to societies which do not share these values. To make the point more emphatically, the author has argued that the academic discipline of psychology itself is heavily eurocentric (although the phenomenon of 'psychology' is not) and that non-Europeans, who carelessly embrace academic psychology without appreciating that it, in many instances, delegitimises their own ethnic psychology, disempower themselves.

Whereas the classical European model of health promotion is predicated as evolving through the individual gaining sufficient self-esteem to work with others (neighbourhood advocacy) and sufficient autonomy to arrive at his or her own health agenda and then negotiating with such authorities as the police, local council, social workers, etc., to realise a community health initiative, none of this would be relevant in most third-world societies. For one thing most societies are compelled by poverty to be highly authoritarian and to de-emphasise individual autonomy.

Cuba provides an interesting example and a counter example. It is a small, poor, third-world nation under authoritarian rule. The difference is that it had a socialist revolution in 1959, replacing a corrupt dictatorship with a communist regime. Among third-world nations it stands out, as far as health is concerned, in that its people may belong to the third world in economic terms, but they die of first-world diseases. Even a cursory study of the epidemiology of most third-world societies shows that the death rates in the first five years of life are much higher than is characteristic in the first world. Also most of these deaths come about through malnutrition, diarrhoea (dehydration) and parasitic disorders. Cuba's socialist system is such that these three have all been largely eliminated, making its epidemiological profile closer to that of the USA and the UK than to that of other third-world nations.

It is interesting to note that health promotion in Cuba was brought about quite differently from what our eurocentric view of health promotion would lead us to believe was the necessary sequence of steps. As the author describes in a paper given at the International Conference on Human Services held at Cambridge in 1996, personal autonomy and the establishment of health agendas through neighbourhood activity played their role in Cuba *after* inter-sectorality had been imposed from above. If health promotion is to become global, it must become a feature of the third world. However, it may well be that the eurocentric model might be the means by which it is achieved. In this they will be more likely to follow the Cuban example.

5

BIOMEDICINE AND HEALTH PROMOTION IN BRITAIN

Globality of the biomedical model

As we saw in Chapter 4, health promotion should be global, but is constrained by many economic and psychological factors in trying to be so. One tendency is for proponents of health promotion to try to define themselves into universality. The reader will appreciate that a number of contemporary models of health promotion exist (see Naidoo and Wills 1994, for instance), and some of them are so inclusive in their remit that they almost cast health promotion in the role of being what any ideologue says it ought to be. As we have seen, the concept of 'empowerment' is likewise carelessly handled in that it can be taken to mean whatever current ideology dictates. Such nebulosity in the use of terms, rather than protecting the integrity of the philosophy and principles of health promotion, renders it unassessable in the NHS except in terms of the criteria of the biomedical model.

In 1995, R. Cook pointed out that health promotion in the NHS had truly become medicalised. The recent spate of healthcare reforms has seen health promotion increasingly ensconced within the NHS, rather than outside of it (Naidoo and Wills 1994). But the NHS, as a bastion of medicine, has very limited ability to tackle the wider determinants of health (Moran 1991). Despite this, GPs, as providers of NHS services to the community, are being sponsored to provide medically-orientated health promotion services. Medicalisation of health promotion represents a narrow conceptualisation of health, for it sees health as occurring within, and being the responsibility of the individual. This is victim-blaming by any other name. Health promotion within the medical model is directed toward the individual without always attempting to address the wider socio-economic and environmental determinants of that person's health. Indeed, medical models of health promotion could more properly be called the medical models of disease prevention and of health education. To that extent, it can be regarded as a limited subset of wider, more socially-orientated health promotion activity.

When one considers the philosophical, cognitive and methodological differences between the scope of medicine and the various activities required to improve people's health by improving their socio-economic and environmental circumstances, the putative placement of health promotion within the health service requires exploration. This chapter will consider the roles or parts played by the major players, the medical profession and the state, in the positioning of the medicine and health promotion. The discussion will therefore consider the power held by these players in relation to each other, as well as to 'minor' players, socially-orientated health promoters and individuals.

Health promotion, particularly in the UK, is critically analysed, and the nature of this activity is then compared with the broader, socially-orientated health promotion as described by the WHO. An explanation is given of the medical model of health and its general acceptance through the rise of medicine and the nature of the medical profession. Consideration is then accorded the power of doctors in society. The relationship between medicine and the state is then explored and is represented in the model of countervailing powers. This allows the relationship between medicine, the state, individuals and socially-orientated health promoters to be set out.

It will be argued in this chapter that, in the UK, the current positioning of medicine and health promotion activity arises from the nature of the medical profession, and its relationship with the state. That is, the values and characteristics of medicine have shaped its social and political standing, and thus determined its actual relationship with the state. This process of contested power-sharing between medicine and the state has brought about the current position of medicine as a vehicle for legitimising the stated objective of promoting individual responsibility for health, bringing us face-to-face once more with the phenomenon of victim blaming.

Health promotion as handmaiden to the NHS

It has already been observed that the Health Service reforms between 1986 and 1996 have increasingly placed health promotion activity within the NHS, rather that outside of it (Naidoo and Wills 1994). Under the new reforms, GPs are expected, as independent contractors providing NHS services to the community, to provide a range of health 'promotion' services (Yen 1995; Allsop 1995) and have been nominated by the Government to do so. Within medical practice, health promotion concentrated on individuals and their behaviour in determining their own health. As the reader knows, purely medical interventions can be divided into three levels: primary healthcare; secondary healthcare; and tertiary healthcare. Primary healthcare uses strategies to prevent the onset of disease, such as mass immunisation programmes. Secondary healthcare activities concentrate on early medical intervention to limit or control disease processes by screening for risk factors or the presence of pre-symptomatic disease. Tertiary healthcare involves minimising the effects of already-established disease (Jones 1994; Naidoo and Wills 1994).

But changes to GP contracts in 1991 and 1993 have reorientated the emphasis of GP work from cure to prevention, by providing financial incentives. Thus the 1991 changes reduced GPs' overall capitation fees, while increasing payments for a broad range of preventive activity (Cook 1995). Yen (1995) points out that, at a time of financial austerity in the NHS, GPs had an open-ended budget for a range of preventive interventions. Changes introduced in 1993 narrowed the spectrum of the activity to concentrate on specific targets, primarily coronary heart disease (CHD) (Cook 1995). The incorporation of a system rendered it possible to rank the nature of, and the remuneration for, interventions to reduce the risks and incidence of CHD. It is now the case that fiscal resources, and therefore activities, are directed toward the individual – to identifying people 'at risk' of heart disease and persuading them to be more responsible for their own health by changing their behaviour so as to prevent heart disease.

Alongside these changes to GP activities, the role of the Health Education Authority (HEA) and community health teams are also being redirected to support primary healthcare team activity. Proposals which allow GPs to directly employ health visitors and community nurses would mean that these professionals will come under medical control to help meet medically-orientated objectives (Cowley 1995; Cole 1996). It is therefore an unquestionable fact that the future of health promotion appears to be becoming progressively more medically-orientated (Cook 1995).

Consequences of the commodity model

As will be discussed more fully in the final chapter of this book, many problems arise when we try to objectify 'health' as a 'commodity' and then to make its promotion the focus of 'targets', 'aims', 'objectives', 'performance indicators' and the like. 'Health' would be complex enough if it only included measurable clinical criteria. Let us just briefly consider that proposition. Suppose in some measurable way we could regard clinical health as a commodity of the classical 'guns' or 'butter' type beloved of economic theorists. Even under those circumstances we would encounter immense difficulties in evaluating attempts to 'promote' it, or even to decide on criteria for doing so, because of the essentially elastic time-scale that we would have to use. For instance, the expense involved in infancy immunisation programmes might have a measurable effect at the other end of a person's life-span and with no clear certainty, when the investment was made, as to when that would be.

But really, of course, the problem is much more involved than that, because 'health' is not confined to clinically measured criteria. It involves all sorts of imponderably abstract qualities, such as feelings of self-esteem, capacity for optimism, even a sense of humour. All of these factors, and many others, certainly make an impact on 'clinical health' and, to add to the labyrinthine complexity, vice versa. Only if we obdurately insist that health is purely a consequence of measurable forces and that healthcare practice is made up of a correspondingly complementary set of measurable forces, does 'health promotion' appear even remotely targetable as a subject for academic discourse. One uncomfortable result of this is that many do, in fact, regard health promotion in exactly that light, not because that model reflects reality, but because it renders it easier to administer.

The author, not only refutes that limited model, but invites the reader to consider the unfortunate consequences of using 'health promotion' as a sort of etymological 'hold all' for any health related consideration that does not easily fit into any other category and, accordingly, seems resolutely to resist empirical analysis. In considering this, the word 'global' instantly springs to this author's mind, not only in the sense of meaning 'world-wide' but in the sense of being 'all things to all people', wherever they are.

Continued use of the phrase 'health promotion' in that sense threatens, this author argues, to rob it of any analytical validity. Once it falls into that category, then it will become a simple matter to equivocate on, say, the very real social consequences of empowerment, neighbourhood advocacy and the like. The medicalisation of health promotion in the embrace of the NHS is only one of a variety of possible consequences of acquiescing in its 'globalisation'.

The singling out of individuals as targets of health promotion represents an exceedingly narrow interpretation of health promotion activity as described by the WHO. In 1974 Marc Lalonde, the Canadian Minister for Health, described health as the product of man's biology, his lifestyle, his environment and the healthcare system to which he had access (Lalonde 1974). It is not widely appreciated that it was really his conceptualisation of health that provided the foundations for the WHO strategies for improving universal health by the year 2000, outlined in Alma Alta in 1978 and in the Ottawa Charter in 1986 and to which Britain was a signatory (Naidoo and Wills 1994).

Strategies were sought for improving health for all including activities to address those areas of life over which individuals had, at the most, only limited control, but which affected their health, and which the state managed on their behalf. At Alma Alta all participating governments became signatories to an agreement to assist individuals to make healthy choices easy choices. This was to be accomplished by considering the impact of all aspects of state activity on the health of its population. For instance, social models of health promotion share a set of values and guiding principles that reflect a more holistic concept of the individual, and acknowledge the social, economic and environmental influences on health. Approaches by such agencies to health promotion are guided by principles of empowerment, community participation, equity in health, accountability, and co-operation and partnership with other agencies and sectors (Naidoo and Wills 1994).

Such an enterprise emphasises the need for health authorities, government agencies, voluntary and commercial organisations to work together to facilitate and promote healthy lifestyles.

All social models of health promotion include targets for disease reduction, they do not abandon the medical model of health promotion but add to it a greater concern for the social and environmental framework within which health and ill-health arise (Jones 1994). This would indicate that the greater part of health promotion activity should lie outside the scope of the NHS.

The medical approach to health promotion often focuses on the individual and attempts to reshape individual behaviour without adequately addressing socio-economic and environmental factors that contribute either to behaviour or to health. Medicalisation in the field of health promotion can be related, in part, to the characteristics of the medical model of health, and the particular set of values associated with medicine and the medical profession. It is a truism that that model has dominated the healthcare professional's, and to some extent the community's, perception of health for the last 150 years (Jones 1994).

The rise of the medical model

As we have already observed, the medical model of health arose as part of the general development of science and of medicine as a profession. But these have to be seen as two distinct issues, as shall now be explained. The period of Enlightenment presented new ways of thinking about and interpreting the nature of the world. Deductive scientific approaches appeared to offer new ways of understanding natural phenomena through deconstruction, observation and interpretation. Simultaneously, there was a gradual relaxation of the church's prohibition of human dissection and anatomical study, and a period of discovery ensued. Dissection of human corpses provided structural and functional information about the body. An 'anatomical atlas' was developed, which provided a new way of seeing and understanding the human body, referred to by Foucault as the 'clinical gaze' (Jones 1994).

Starting at the University of Padua in about 1540, dissection facilitated the collection of knowledge about what was clinically normal and abnormal. Empirical and non-religiously based information about what was 'normal' consequently reorientated thinking about disease. Associated with 'normal' structure and function was 'health', and, therefore, 'disease' was that which was observed to arise when structure and/or function were abnormal. All disease could, in theory, be explained in biological terms. For disease to occur within the individual, that individual must have brought it about by 'bad' behaviour. Due to great increases in knowledge and the appreciation of discoveries in physics, a mechanistic view of the body emerged. Illness was now envisaged as affecting a particular body organ, rather that the whole person, and treatment was directed at the abnormal body part (Jones 1994; Naidoo and Wills 1994).

Naturally enough, these characteristics of the medical model of health are faithfully reflected in the medical model of health promotion. If it is held that health is equated with functional fitness and the absence of disease, health promotion activities ought to be directed toward prevention, cure and limitation of specific illnesses. We can use scientific and medical interventions, it would seem, to achieve these aims, and such interventions are directed toward the individual. Indeed, if disease processes take place within the individual, it should be feasible to teach people how they can modify their behaviour to prevent or limit disease processes.

Authority of the medical profession

Although the foregoing description provides an adequate rationale for the gradual emergence of biomedicine as a successful model for coping with illness, it must be appreciated that another factor was involved. The practitioners of medicine obviously were also proactive in arrogating power to themselves. The more they did this, and the more convincingly they did it, not least because they believed themselves to be right, the more people were ready and willing to hand over responsibility for their health to them. Thus a large part of the general acceptance of the medical view of health and illness must be attributed to the power of the medical profession (Jones 1994). The characteristics of a profession, as described by Freidson (1970), go some way toward explaining that power.

Freidson identifies autonomy as the distinguishing characteristic of a profession. This autonomy, that is control over the content and terms of work, is associated with the possession of expert knowledge. In turn, the power of a professional group is related to its control over expert knowledge and this confers on it leverage over any person or group who needs that expertise. Such groups preserve themselves and the nature of a professional group is such that its activities are in part directed toward the maintenance of its powerful position within society. It is also the case that a profession controls expert information by restricting access to that information; by directing its activity toward furthering its body of expert knowledge and by maintaining itself as the only one able to interpret that expert knowledge to the unknowing. Through thus controlling information, a profession is in a position to dominate the division of labour and organisation of services so as to facilitate the advancement of its own goals (Freidson 1970).

Prior to the rise of scientific medicine, of course, the UK enjoyed several 'models' of health and consequently generated a myriad of healthcare practitioners. Theories of health such as the miasma theory and humoral theory were widely accepted (Jones 1994; Donaldson and Donaldson 1993). But scientific medicine did have the advantage of being able to predict, even if it could not effectively treat, illness (Jones 1994). This placed doctors, as a developing profession, in a powerful position and they exploited it.

Increasingly, people looked to the scientific approach and other healthcare workers and alternative models of health were successfully subjugated. The Medical Registration Act of 1858 effectively eliminated all other contenders in the sphere of healthcare (Jones 1994; Larkin 1995).

Towards the end of the nineteenth century, the medical profession was on the way to becoming successful and recognised as being 'legitimate', by riding on the prestige of scientific and biological breakthroughs. This subsequently made its medical monopoly more credible (Richman 1987).

Analysis of eighteenth- and nineteenth-century health statistics has revealed that public health measures contributed more to eighteenth-century health than clinical medicine had (McKeown 1979). Public health reforms such as improved sanitation and water supplies led to vast improvements in life chances. It is interesting that many of these reforms were underpinned by quite egregiously defective 'scientific' theories. For instance, the miasma theory, which held that disease came about by bad smells arising from putre-faction, sewage, etc., led to underground sewerage piping, etc. This made a significant and lasting improvement to health, even though the theory behind it was so wrong (Jones 1994; Donaldson and Donaldson 1994). The Royal Sanitary Commission produced a report which led to the establishment of a central department of public health, with local authorities employing medical officers of health (National Association of Health Authorities and Trusts (NAHAT) 1995/6).

Initially public health and medicine were two discrete entities. This remained the case until the advent of germ theory in the late nineteenth century challenged the miasma theory that had underpinned public health initiatives. Germ theory refocused attention on the body, and the organisms that invaded it, in causing disease (Jones 1994).

Large-scale intervention, through public health, and with the intention of improving the local environment, gave way to public health as a medically controlled enterprise. This called for study, guidance and control of the individual. In particular, the germ theory brought people's lives under a now extended clinical gaze, and engendered an attack on personal habits and hygiene (Jones 1994).

It has been suggested (Moran 1991) that the fundamental difference between public health and general medicine is that the public is concerned with collective health, while medicine is concerned with that of individuals. Upon the formation of the NHS, public health remained under local authority control while curative medicine moved forward under the NHS (Moran 1991). It is also true that the NHS reforms of the 1970s increased the distance between medicine and public and environmental health. This reorganisation left the NHS as a purely individualist-focused, medically orientated service (Moran and Watkins 1991).

51

The NHS's role

At the time when the NHS came into being (1948) the hospital was regarded as the pinnacle of medical science. The specialist, because he had expertise, was in a position to control the work and resources to meet his own objectives. In this way the value of scientific advancement and of the medical expert shaped the role of the hospital (Jones 1994). In turn, the organisation of other hospital personnel was directed toward meeting the needs of the consultants, and their professional training often followed the medical model of health (Caraher 1994; Jones 1994). In this context, GPs referred problematic patients to specialists in hospitals, the hub of medical care and centre of excellence (Calnan and Williams 1995). Accordingly, as the hospital expert channelled resources into scientific advancement, the distance between hospital medicine and general practice grew.

For many years, the role of the GP has centred on preventive medicine and specifically on the limitation of chronic disease (Cook 1995). The medical profession itself has developed and enhanced this. By the 1950s the BMS was portraying GPs as specialising in continuous and preventive care so that in the 1970s general practice had come to be regarded as the natural home of health education (Calnan *et al.* 1986).

From its inception the Royal College of General Practitioners (RCGP) has emphasised the role of GPs in illness prevention. Specifically in the early 1980s they detailed such appropriate activities as: pre-symptom screening; opportunistic preventive education for patients presenting in surgery; and greater involvement in 'community' activities, such as working with teachers to educate children about, for example, 'relationships' or 'sexual love and childbirth' (Calnan *et al.* 1986). Of course, much of the impetus behind the RCGP statement came from practitioners themselves and has been interpreted as an attempt by GPs to enhance and maintain a professional identity that was independent of hospital medicine (Calnan *et al.* 1986).

Advances in medicine and of the medical profession have had far-reaching effects, both for individuals and their communities. The medical model of health has shaped people's perception of health and illness, and has altered their ability to deal with illness.

Obviously the relationship between patient and doctor is weighted in favour of the latter because he/she holds esoteric knowledge which has to be interpreted for the layman. Patient opinion is subservient to that of the doctor whose specialist knowledge can be used to determine what is best for the patient (Freidson 1970).

Illich (1979) was concerned about the impact of medicine on society. He saw the dependency of the patient on his doctor as being detrimental to both the individual and to society. Through cultivating a dependence of the patient on medical expertise, the doctor was inadvertently contributing to the breakdown of social and cultural ways of coping with life issues such as birth and death.

The earlier example of GPs becoming involved in teaching school children about relationships typifies what Zola referred to as the creeping
medicalisation of everyday life (Zola 1975). Zola contended that if anything
could be shown in some way to adversely affect the workings of the body or
mind then it could be labelled an 'illness' or 'a medical problem' (1975). In that
way, medicine, because it is concerned with the wellbeing of individuals, can
intrude upon any aspect of everyday life it perceives as affecting health. No
exaggeration is required to suggest that, by logical extension, anything that
affects future health also falls within its remit.

The power and persuasion of the medical profession is now such that
medical evidence and rhetoric may be used to advance any cause seen as
relevant to the good practice of medicine (Jones 1994). Likewise, since medicine
strives to prevent illness and promote health, it can legitimately become
involved in any aspect of individual lifestyles that affect health or future health.
It is therefore not difficult to be beguiled by the argument that the medical
approach to health promotion is not only justified, but is necessary for the
good of the individual. From such a perspective one can see that legitimately
becoming extended to include the surveillance of the lives of well people.

Medicalisation as an identifiable social force

We have, then, so far accounted for how and why the institution of medicine
has assumed the form of a discrete and powerful entity that has monopolised
healthcare and had a profound impact on society. The nature of the medical
profession is such that it has maintained control over expert knowledge and
has shaped healthcare to such an extent that the utilisation of resources is
directed toward the advancement of its own expertise. Through this development, the dependence of the layman for interpretation and judgement is
assured and medicine has extended its practice into the realms of everyday life
for the good of the patient.

Of course, medicalisation has been criticised from several angles. For
example, its conceptualisation of health has been challenged for its individualist approach. Already a number of health promoters have become
concerned with the medical model of health promotion's domination of
health promotion activity, given its narrow conception of factors affecting
health and illness (Allsop 1995; Jones 1994; Moran 1991). As well, the medical
profession's domination of healthcare and its refusal to share power with
other professionals has been criticised (Jones 1994). Feminist critiques are
particularly important in challenging the partial domination of women as a
social construct to facilitate their subservience in social and professional roles
(Oakley 1984; Savage 1986; Miles 1991). In its wider impact on society, both at
individual and community level, medicine has been interpreted as either
incidental or instrumental in assuring the future of medicine (Zola 1975; Illich
1979; Navarro 1976).

It is with the power of medicine that all these critics are concerned, with its use, misuse or misappropriation. But, as we know, guiding principles of social models of health promotion include empowerment, community participation, co-operation and partnership and all these principles relate to the equitable sharing of power.

Having accounted for medicine's immense power and prestige, it will now be placed in context of the state, where its power can be seen as relative and conditional. It is evident that the basis of power for any body or organisation resides in having a key resource that another organisation or body wants. In general, the properties or resources equated with power-holding are information, expertise or money (Walt 1994). In liberal democracies, leverage is dependent upon who holds which resource and who needs it. It is the retention of expertise which is what both defined the medical profession and gave it leverage in its relationship with the state, according to Freidson (1970).

The concept of medical autonomy has been suggested by Foucault as being part of the process of state formation, for he saw the development of medicine as a profession as an integral part of the development of the state (Johnson *et al.* 1995; Jones 1994). Again, it is government's role to license professional expertise as part of a general process of implementing government objectives and standardising procedures (Johnson *et al.* 1995). Thus, by institutionalising expertise, the government both legitimatises the profession and its own objectives simultaneously. At the same time the stance of the profession is demonstrated to be strictly apolitical (Klein 1984; Johnson *et al.* 1995). This, according to Johnson *et al.*, is because governments depend on the myth of the neutrality of expertise in rendering social realities governable (1995).

The conceptual framework of countervailing powers which can be used to describe profession–state relations has been examined by Light (1995). This framework focuses attention on the interactions of the powerful players in a field where they are inherently interactive while yet distinct. A fair distribution of power is feasible and desirable and if one party dominates or over-exploits the power base, then a counteraction by the other player(s) ensues. These countermoves strive to redress the imbalance of power rather than to destroy the dominant player.

We observe that in those states in which the government has played a central role in nurturing professions within the state structure, but has allowed the professions to establish their own institutions and power base, the professions and the state will go through phases of harmony and discord in which these countervailing actions take place. That is, dominance by one player slowly produces imbalances that provoke other countervailing (latent) powers to respond. In the process, countervailing powers may attempt to portray benefits to themselves as benefits for everyone, or to portray themselves as victims of other powers and organisations, particularly the state.

Contextually, then, the degree of power consists of one's ability to override, suppress or render irrelevant the challenges by others (Light 1995). By using

Light's framework of countervailing powers, and incorporating the power resources of information, money and expertise, we can portray the relationships between the major players (the medical profession and the state), and thus the relative positions of the minor players (socially-orientated health promoters and individuals).

State versus medicine

Since the end of the Second World War there has been a political consensus about the role of the state in providing for the welfare of its citizens. For instance, it is now accepted that certain people have health and welfare needs, and that the state should allocate and co-ordinate the provision of resources to meet these needs (Walt 1994; Alaszewski 1995). The medical profession had already established itself as the only legitimate body with the expertise to provide this healthcare, and as such it was essential to the state. At the same time, the medical profession had no desire to come under state, and particularly local government, control (Jones 1994). One interpretation of their incentive to participate in the national scheme was to gain access to the key resource of money. In this context, we can speculate that the formation of the NHS represented a deal between the medical profession and the state that called for compromises on both parts yet remained broadly in a line with the objectives of both parties (Jones 1994).

To the present day the medical profession was central to the system of allocating resources, and their expertise and professional objectivity has been relied upon by the government. They had the confidence of the public and were thus positioned as the neutral agents for the fair allocation of resources (Alaszewski 1995).

Over time, an imbalance has arisen as the medical profession consumed more and more of the government's resources, and became more powerful with it. As a countervailing action, the state attempted to curb the resources available to medicine, for example by the introduction of a restricted pharmaceutical list, and of general management initiatives (Walt 1994).

But the power of the medical profession, and particularly its social standing, remains such that the state cannot challenge medicine without provoking a countervailing action that presents the state's motives as suspect (Light 1995). Therefore, in order to render challenges to the power of medicine socially acceptable, the state has consistently portrayed the medical profession as being profligate with tax-payer's money (Walt 1994).

The fundamental shift in power came with the breakdown in consensus of the state's role in providing healthcare (Walt 1994). Obviously, consensual power sharing is dependent upon both parties having something that the other needs and the underlying strength in the medical profession's position was that the state had accepted responsibility for the health of the nation, and that the medical profession was central to delivering healthcare (Alaszewski

1995). It can be argued that the breakdown in consensus of the state's role and obligations in the provision of comprehensive healthcare undermined the leverage of medicine (Walt 1994).

One effect, and an intended one, of the healthcare reforms of the 1980s was a redistribution and dissemination of power within the medical profession. This has changed the power relationship between the profession and the state (Allsop 1995).

We can see that the introduction of managerial principles, particularly accountability, challenged the previously free hand of the specialist in controlling resources (Calnan and Williams 1995). Again, the separation of purchasers and providers of healthcare, and the introduction of GP fundholding, repositioned power within the medical profession. Consultants were now accountable to managers, who were increasingly able to control consultants' work and remuneration. In the broader community, GP fundholding status served to increase the standing of GPs in relation to hospital consultants (Loewenberg 1996; Calnan and Williams 1995). But for the GPs, the increased autonomy that came with holding their own budgets was tempered with their subservience to the Family Health Service Authority (FHSA) (Allsop 1995; Calnan and Williams 1995).

This widespread reorientating of power within the medical profession has theoretically shifted the financial resources and therefore the power away from the hospital and into the community. The government has attempted to present this as an attempt at community empowerment that [rightly] refocused medical perception of the patient as a member of a community (Alaszewski 1995). For the state itself the benefit was a legitimate curtailment of spiralling hospital costs and consequently of specialist power (Naidoo and Wills 1994; Allsop 1995).

It has been contended (Walt 1994) that the medical profession has been relegated from a privileged position as a player at the centre of health policymaking to a rather more marginal position as a sectional interest or pressure group. Its position as a countervailing power has certainly been seriously undermined.

Now the dominance of resources by the medical profession has been effectively challenged by the state, representing a countervailing action from one major player against another. The foundation of the power-sharing relationship between medicine and state has been undermined, and the power within the medical profession has accordingly been redistributed.

It is when the powers of socially-orientated health promoters and individuals are applied to the countervailing framework that their status can be seen as peripheral to both medicine and the state. To be seen as constituting an effective countervailing power, a body or organisation must hold at least one resource. However, neither socially-orientated health promoters nor individuals hold any resource that the major players want. Whatever challenge they make can be effectively suppressed, ignored or rendered irrelevant, regardless of its validity, simply because it is not backed by a power-giving resource.

The various critics of the medical models of health have come to the fore as countervailing groups, purely in response to the dominance of medicine, and of its impact on society. Perceptions of imbalance as perceived by the critics, were related to medicine's reluctance to share power with other healthcare professionals, rather than with its construction of health (Jones 1994). Moreover, such challenges have had little significant impact on the provision of healthcare (Savage 1986; Jones 1994).

However, while it is true that socially-orientated health promoters do not hold any key resource, the fundamental principles of social models may be seen by both medicine and government as having broad support, and are therefore useful. The rhetoric of social models may be used by both state and medicine to their own advantage, without adopting the basic tenets. In this manner government may claim that healthcare should be centred in the community to facilitate community empowerment, but their actions do not facilitate real empowerment, and its being placed there has strong advantages for government. Similarly, medicine may denounce complementary practice as ineffective, but it suits medicine to suppress the competition, while representing itself as a benevolent guardian of the nation's welfare (Larkin 1995).

Accounting for the present state of affairs

Foucault's concept that the state's relationship with professions is both to legitimise and apply its objectives, is still pertinent (Johnson 1995). While thus reducing the power of medicine, the values of the medical model and the credibility afforded by the medical profession can be used to advance and legitimise the government objective of increasing the individual's own responsibility for his health (Allsop 1995).

The foregoing analysis renders the New Right philosophy of individualism entirely compatible with the medical model's conception of health. Accommodating easily with behavioural and lifestyle-focused health promotion initiatives, it allows people to be held responsible for their own health. It suggests to them that they can, with changes to their behaviour, become healthy (Baum and Saunders 1995).

Today, with the medical profession under financial control, the state is, for the first time, in a position to shape that nature of the medical work. So far interventions are directed toward enhancing medicine's individualist and behaviourist conceptions of health, but this can change with social policy. We have seen that in the 1991 reforms, the state gave GPs clear incentives and financial scope to develop the medical model of health promotion.

In 1993 the new contracts took a fundamentally more controlling approach. Weighting of funding for different bands of interventions at present indicate a more concerted move toward identification and management of risk factors

(Cook 1995). Some see this as representing an increasingly pervasive managerialist approach for both professions and consumers (Yen 1995; Allsop 1995). For instance, increased emphasis on identification of risk factors effectively extends the GP's and consequently the state's authority over the well population. It becomes the purpose of screening to detect those 'at risk' so that they can be counselled about lifestyles, thereby extending clinical surveillance of the lives of the well population. The scientific authority of medicine and of medical technology legitimises claims about the advantages of early detection and treatment, thus ensuring patient compliance. Finally, medical compliance is ensured through financial incentives (Allsop 1995).

At Alma Alta, primary healthcare (PHC) was identified as the key to achieving Health for All by the year 2000. Initially this definition of PHC anticipated a comprehensive approach improving communities' and individuals' health status. From the outset it stressed the importance of access to community-based services that place emphasis on prevention and action outside the health sector to promote health (Baum and Saunders 1995).

It is not difficult to appreciate, therefore, that there is a considerable distance between the comprehensive strategies outlined in Alma Alta and the current selective and targeted approach to disease control. Promoting selective primary healthcare interventions under the PHC umbrella has had the effect of retaining intervention firmly within medical control and therefore of state control. Therefore, the placement of health promotion within medicine serves to detract from the need for longer-term social, economic and political change (Farrant 1991).

6

THE 'HEALTH OF THE NATION' TARGETS AND HEALTH PROMOTION

The White Paper

The Government's White Paper, *The Health of the Nation,* was finally published in July 1992. It followed on from the Green Paper which had been produced the previous year to allow a period of consultation from experts and interested lay groups. The response to the Green Paper had been enthusiastic and had provoked much publicity and debate, particularly among the medical and nursing professions. The *British Medical Journal* ran a four-month series of letters and articles on the details of the proposals (*BMJ*, July–October 1991).

In discussing the implications of this document for the future of health policy in England and its claims to offer a viable strategy for health and health promotion, it is important to provide some insight into the contemporary influences and political situation. Both of these very much contributed to the formulation of a policy which, at least in appearance, constituted such a radical departure from other health policies of the time.

It is necessary also to appraise critically the strategy being proposed in the White Paper in the context of the debate surrounding health promotion. It is then possible to draw some conclusions as to whether the White Paper did provide a truly viable strategy for achieving the targets and the overall improvements in the nation's health, which it proposed to do.

The Health of the Nation White Paper was the first ever government policy in Britain that provided a strategy for the future health of the nation and this in itself secures for it a unique position in the context of health policy in Britain. Its importance should not be underestimated.

A foundation for health promotion internationally

The rationale for producing a strategy for health had developed from the work of the WHO. The WHO had convened a number of key conferences during the 1970s and 1980s to promote discussion on the issues of health for all nations. The ideas, structure and strategy for *The Health of the Nation* stemmed directly from the ideas being expressed by the WHO at this time and involved principally a move away from a medically determined model of healthcare towards the multidisciplinary concept of health promotion.

The WHO followed on from its international conference at Alma Ata in 1978, producing its Health for All strategy in 1981. The main importance of the WHO *Health for All* document was in offering the idea of a 'strategy for health' based on the principles of 'target setting'. This also forms the core of the Government's proposals, indeed the actual full title of *The Health of the Nation* includes the phrase *A Strategy for Health in England*. The means by which the strategy would be attained was in the setting of specific targets in nominated 'key areas', many of which were the same in the two documents including the target areas for cancers, heart disease and stroke, accidents and suicide (WHO 1981; Department of Health (DOH) 1992).

The language of the two documents also had similarities. The *Health for All* document proposed 'adding life to years' and 'adding health to life', phrases mirrored in *The Health of the Nation* which talked of 'adding years to life' and 'adding life to years' (DOH 1992). The WHO document was also fundamental in its recognition of the millennium, the year 2000, as a beacon for its targets, the time-scale on which most of *The Health of the Nation* targets were also set.

There were a number of other areas in which *The Health of the Nation* proposals have been influenced by the work of the WHO. The issuance of the Ottawa Charter, for example, in 1986 was important in its identification of the principles of health promotion, rather than a medically determined model of disease diagnosis and treatment, as an objective for future global health policy. There was a newly determined emphasis on the importance of 'healthy public policy' as a prerequisite for improvements in the health of populations. At the heart of successful public policy was the need to establish strong communities, to forge alliances among different interested bodies and to eradicate poverty and social injustice (WHO 1986).

The Health of the Nation accepted much of the discourse on these issues as fundamental to its own strategy (Parish 1991). In its formulation of a national strategy as a 'healthy public policy', in its recognition of the need for the participation of communities and in its objectives to establish 'healthy alliances' (DOH 1992), it did indeed appear to have caught the thrust of the WHO initiative and especially of the Ottawa Charter.

As some writers have pointed out, there does appear to be a degree of selectivity or at least a dilution of much of the radical ideas emanating from the WHO and the actual strategies contained in *The Health of the Nation* (Gray 1991; Radical Statistics Health Group 1991a, 1991b; Wilkinson 1995).

Attempts to avoid a social agenda

This is perhaps best illustrated by the divergence in emphasis between the

WHO and the White Paper on issues such as poverty, social injustice and the environment. These are seen as fundamental to health promotion by the WHO, but are relegated to a back seat compared to the importance of individual lifestyle and increased efficiency of health service provision. The White Paper also reflects strong leanings towards cost effectiveness (Radical Statistics Health Group 1991a, 1991b; Whitehead 1992; Wilkinson 1995). Indeed why should a government which had steadfastly ignored the findings of its own investigation into inequalities in health, published in the Black Report 1989, suddenly find so much truth in the recommendations of the WHO on issues such as these? These very important considerations have been mentioned here but are referred to again in the more detailed analysis of the proposed strategy and its viability as a tool for health promotion.

In offering a degree of discussion around the concepts and international pressures for change which informed *The Health of the Nation* document, it is important not to ignore the domestic political atmosphere which may also have influenced Government policy. There is some debate as to why the Government should have adopted such a strategy at all and one which at face value appeared to owe so much to an organisation not noted for its high-profile with the British Government, a government which liked to dismiss outside influence as interference.

One possibility for the apparent change in strategy was to offer a spoonful of sugar with which to help the nation swallow the bitter pill of the earlier health reforms (the 1990 Health Service and Community Care Act) (Radical Statistics Health Group 1991a, 1991b; Butler 1993). The Government had found to its cost, in terms of its popularity, the dangers of tampering with the much beloved National Health Service. They had indeed even been forced to tone down much of the original language contained in these reforms in order to offset growing hostility (Sheldon 1990; Butler 1993).

Another embarrassment for the Government which may have provoked the need for a change in emphasis was the growing realisation that Britain was faring badly in comparison with other countries on many key health indicators, such as infant mortality, male life expectancy, infertility, and even in comparative rates of survival for cancer sufferers. The National Health Service was failing to keep up with the rising expectations of the nation and a policy that enabled the Government to shift the emphasis away from hospital-based medical services towards the community was seen as potentially beneficial (Ham 1993; Butler 1993).

The final draft of the Government's White Paper was published in July 1992 and followed on from the Green Paper and the consultation period of the previous year. The final strategy is summarised in the White Paper in five main points: the selection of five key areas for action; the setting of the national objectives and targets in these key areas; indications for the action required to achieve the targets; an outline of the initiative to aid in implementation of the strategy; and the setting up of a framework for monitoring, development and review (DOH 1992).

Analysis of the five points of strategy

These five points constitute the basis of the entire strategy and in order to form any basis for analysis they must be examined fully in terms of their implications for health promotion.

The Green Paper originally proposed sixteen potential key areas for action, but these were eventually reduced to five for the White Paper. The selection was based on the principle that the areas would establish the idea of a clear set of priorities for intervention in areas of the greatest need and where there was sufficient scope to bring about cost-effective improvements in health across the country (DOH 1992). The key areas had to have been shown to be a major cause of premature death (a death under the age of sixty-five), or avoidable ill health, and to offer the possibility of 'measurable and achievable' targets.

The five key areas eventually selected were: coronary heart disease and stroke; cancers; mental illness; HIV/AIDS and sexual health; and accidents. Those which were eventually rejected included a strategy for asthma, the ageing population, child health, pregnant women and alcohol. There was a considerable degree of criticism levied at the strategy for the exclusion of these as key areas. It had been suggested, for example, that the elderly may have been cynically omitted as a key area on the basis that they are a broadly politically inactive group and therefore pose no threat to Government popularity by their exclusion (Grimley Evans 1991). In the light of recent evidence about the demographics of an ageing population, the future health needs of this particular group would seem to warrant special attention and it does, therefore, appear to have been a serious omission, even more so in retrospect.

Other criticisms over the exclusion of possible key areas have centred on the fact that many were rejected on the grounds that there was a lack of available data for measurement (Radical Statistics Health Group 1991a, 1991b). The White Paper does not, however, attempt to make a lack of available data a target in itself and areas which were deficient in the relevant quantative data were automatically excluded from the White Paper on these grounds alone.

Questioning the rationale for the targets

The targets in themselves have also been the source of some debate and criticism. Many of the targets, it has been claimed, appear to have been plucked out of the sky (Smith 1991), and therefore seem to be unrealistic. For example, the figures quoted all appear to be round percentages: a reduction in the suicide rate of 15 per cent by the year 2000; a reduction of 40 per cent in the death rates from coronary heart disease and strokes by the year 2000; a reduction of 25 per cent in the death rate from breast cancer again by the year 2000. These targets do not appear to be based on any specific criteria and there is no mention of how these figures have been derived (DOH 1992). One obvious basis for them might be the thirty-eight WHO targets for *Health for All* 2000, in many of which the same sort of 'numerical eclecticism' is evident. This author has argued that much of that comes about through arguing the *relative* merits of targets in committee, so that the percentages arrived at reflect compromises rather than epidemiological criteria.

The validity of much of the target information has also been called into question on the grounds that some of the targets are misleading. For example, the implication of much of the need for target setting in the first instance is that the mortality and morbidity rates in particular areas were rising, thereby creating the need for intervention to bring about the proposed fall. However, in the case of many of the key areas the death rates already appeared to be declining. In the case of heart disease and strokes, this decline was already at a rate which would suggest that the targets would be reached with no further intervention by the Government.

In the case of some of the other targets, criticism has been levelled at the fact that they may have been misleading and irrelevant. The White Paper makes assumptions which have not necessarily been proven, although they may hold popular sway. The association between obesity and ill health, for instance, has never been adequately explained but in the White Paper the association is made out to be very strong, 'obesity acts to increase the risk of CHD and stroke through its association with an increased prevalence of raised blood pressure and raised plasma cholesterol' (DOH 1992).

The focus on mental health

In the targets set for mental illness, the White Paper makes the assumption that the suicide rate reflects the overall rate of mental illness in society and that, by reducing the rates of suicide, the general mental health of the population will be improved. As Charlotte Pearson points out, however:

> A clear link between mental illness and suicide has not been made. Only a proportion of people committing suicide are mentally ill, and a reduction of the suicide rate is not necessarily an efficient measure of the extent of mental health problems.
>
> (Pearson 1992)

Durkheim, in his seminal study of the sociology of suicide in 1870, cautioned against the over simplification of its causes. He also pointed out that suicide rates could only be reduced by changes in society as a whole and not merely by the increased education, repression or exhortation of individuals.

The Government's proposals for reducing suicide are to increase 'information and understanding', particularly among health professionals, in the expectation that potential suicides, might be discovered earlier. In the case of young suicides, however, much evidence suggests that the act is committed impulsively (Hawton 1993; Platt 1989). It is therefore unlikely that much benefit would be gained from increased professional awareness, as this group are not easily identifiable.

Legislative advantages of the targets

Despite the criticism levelled at the White Paper on target setting, it must be said that the selection of five key areas has subsequently allowed for the setting of real priorities. The selected areas are not intended, according to the White Paper, to be an end in themselves but rather to be the beginning of a 'rolling programme' for action (DOH 1992). The idea was that, once targets had been attained, new ones could be set or new target areas prepared.

The setting of targets in selected areas has become a generally accepted method of fixing an agenda and establishing a strategy for health and is in accordance with the directives of the WHO (1981). It is worth noting that the White Paper was received favourably by the WHO for being the first national strategy for health, which took into account some of the recent principles of health promotion. It does appear to make sense that health strategy in Britain should reflect the health agenda being established at an international level (Smith 1991; Garbay 1992).

The Government has aimed at achieving its targets by the establishment of a course of action for each of the key target areas. It is in this aspect of the White Paper that criticism has been the most hard hitting. It is interesting to note, for example, that there is much talk in the White Paper of a strategy for health and health promotion: 'The Government's overall goal is to secure continuing improvement in the general health of the population of England' (DOH 1992). This is to be achieved through the creation of 'high quality health services'.

At no point, however, does the White Paper offer a definition of health on which to base its strategy. This is in spite of the fact that the WHO had already established a working definition of health promotion in 1984 as 'the process of enabling people to increase control over, and to improve, their health'.

Philosophical strategic problems

The failure to establish what is meant by health or health promotion, despite the frequent reference to these terms in the White Paper, has imbued the document with a distinctly biomedical orientation toward health. Health is therefore seen as a purely negative state, a lack of something, of being without disease. Health is seen as being the opposite of illness and, in order to improve, disease must be eradicated.

This in a large part accounts for much of the planned action devised for the White Paper, which is mainly based on increased screening for the early detection of disease. In the strategy for the targets set for cancer reductions, for example, the actions are largely based on a planned increase in the availability and frequency of screening (DOH 1992). Screening as a means of disease prevention is not without its critics, however. Wendy Savage showed that cervical screening was often misunderstood by women. For example, the vast majority (71 per cent) of the women in one study undertaken by her felt that the purpose of cervical screening was to detect cancer, not to prevent it (Savage 1989), and it was this misunderstanding which resulted in the poor uptake of the programme, not a lack of availability.

Screening in itself is a fundamentally medical intervention and is certainly not innovative in terms of preventive medicine. Even in this respect it is seen to have its limitations for, despite the long history and availability of cervical screening, there has never been a significant fall in mortality as a result. There are similar poor statistics for cholesterol measurement and deaths from coronary heart disease, and early breast screening which have not resulted in significant reductions in mortality (Howarth 1991). The over emphasis placed on the importance of such procedures limits many of the White Paper's proposals to means of disease prevention as opposed to real health promotion.

The White Paper establishes the major health problems which require action as being 'avoidable' premature death or disability and what it describes as 'significant variations in ill-health in England as in other countries . . . in different ethnic social and occupational groups and in different geographical regions' (DOH 1992). There has, however, been a great deal of criticism of the White Paper for failing to grasp the real significance of these factors in terms of formulating a strategy for health. For instance, the term 'inequalities in health' has been softened to 'variations in health', possibly a deliberate attempt at distancing it from the terminology and damning evidence of the Report of the Black Commission which had published its findings in 1989 (Mckeown 1995).

Can the targets be politically neutral?

The outline of action in the White Paper also falls short of attempting any structural or economic change, which is regarded by many as an essential prerequisite for the reduction of poverty and social inequalities and their attendant health implications (Townsend and Davidson 1982; WHO 1982, 1984, 1992; Phillimore et al. 1994; Whitehead 1992). Much of the information for the significance of social and economic inequalities on the health and illness of populations was well known at the time of the drawing up of the White Paper (Townsend and Davidson 1982; Marmot 1986; Wilkinson 1986).

The Black Commission had made its report in 1989 and was regarded by many as a well-researched and credible document. It was not, however, favourably received by the Government who at the time took great pains to obscure the report by selective publication and the convenient timing of such publication (Mckeown 1995). There is, therefore, little evidence to suggest that a Government which failed so obviously to acknowledge the findings of its own highly praised commission report could be truly committed to addressing the significance of social inequity in the health debate.

In its lack of commitment to the establishment of a radical policy for healthcare, the White Paper has been accused of falling back on hackneyed rhetoric. Its basic assumption is that health and illness are really determined by individual lifestyle and that, by altering the way we live, health outcomes can be effected. It aims through programmes of health education and exhortation to increase individual responsibility in encouraging people to live healthier lives through sensible eating, increased physical activity, giving up smoking and reducing alcohol consumption.

The 'freedom of choice' argument

There is a very determined belief that people, given enough information by increasing health education initiatives, can 'select' or 'adopt' healthier lifestyles. Implicit in this belief is, however, the notion that if people fail to make the required lifestyle change, they must in some way take responsibility for their own ill-health. This has been criticised as a rather simplistic view of what many now perceive to be the very complex web of interrelated factors which determine health and illness, particularly the part played by socio-economic factors (Townsend and Davidson 1982; WHO 1981, 1984). The White Paper makes no reference at all to the relevance of individual psychology and its relationship to health-related behaviour (Bennett and Murphy 1994).

In its fundamental failure to make explicit the connection between poverty and ill-health and to provide a concerted action plan to reduce social deprivation, it could be argued that much of the strategy for the Health of the Nation has been rendered toothless, lacking in any real power to bring about significant health promotion or disease prevention on a universal level (Gray 1991; Ham 1993; Benzeval *et al.* 1995). Indeed, one effect of this type of strategy may be to broaden the gap because policies based on lifestyle have the least impact in the areas of greatest need, so while an overall improvement in the nation's health may occur, health inequalities will widen as a consequence. What Tudor Hart (1971) termed the 'inverse health law' of those with the greatest need having the least accessibility to healthcare may be exacerbated by the adoption of lifestyle centred health policy.

The need for contextual support

There are a number of other areas of debate concerning the planned action for achieving the targets laid down in *The Health of the Nation* document. The first of these is the accusation that the Government has shied away from adopting significant initiatives in some of the target areas, which may have proved significant in terms of achieving the goals set down, but may well have brought them into conflict with interested groups. This is particularly noticeable in its failure to offer legislation to abolish tobacco advertising.

The prevalence of smoking is referred to in the White Paper as having a significant impact on the incidence of cancers and heart disease and stroke, two of the key areas targeted in the document, and to be a contributory factor in the incidence of avoidable ill-health in the population. In its strategic plan, however, there is no mention of any intention to act punitively towards tobacco manufactures, by making further increases in tobacco tax, or to make provision for a ban on tobacco advertising, even though these factors are well recognised as influencing the prevalence of smoking (DOH 1992). Instead the document confines itself to a plan based on increasing available information to raise awareness of the dangers of smoking and to offering encouragement to people to stop smoking. Both of these policies are already largely in existence and hardly offer anything new (Radical Statistics Health Group 1991a, 1991b).

In its outline for policies related to the environment, the White Paper has been seen to be weak, particularly in its failure to offer any real strategy to tackle pollution, both as a problem in itself and also in establishing the part it plays in health and illness. There are no proposals for an action plan with regards to poor housing or homelessness, although it is accepted, in the White Paper, that the environment is an area over which individuals can have little, if any, real control and therefore the Government is seen as obliged to act on behalf of the public in that arena.

Implementing the targets

Finally it is necessary to look at the organisational strategy for the health of the nation. The Government appears to set great store by co-operation and the formation of healthy alliances in order to adopt a health promotional policy. This is significant in a number of ways. Firstly, it is an attempt to move away from hospital-based medical healthcare towards a more community-centred approach. The White Paper calls for recognition of the potential input from non-professional bodies and of individual members of the public, whose opinions it regards as valuable. This is in keeping with the broader view of health promotion expressed by the WHO and other health promoters, in which the ideas of collaboration are seen to be fundamental to the message of health promotion as being multisectoral and that of the determinants of health as being multifactoral (Nocon 1993).

Despite some genuinely laudable intentions on the issues of collaborative services, the White Paper does not really examine the complexities of forging alliances across numerous disciplines, nor does it offer much in the way of machinery for such effective alliances (Nocon 1993). There are also the potential difficulties raised by the possibility of political conflict, in which a local authority may be under the control of one political party and may find itself unwilling to work with Health Authorities appointed by a Government controlled by another party and implementing government policy, including *The Health of the Nation* (Nocon 1993).

There also exists a contradiction between the new hard-line competition created by market forces and encouragement for team-spirited co-operation (Ewles 1993). In order for any strategy for joint working to become effective, there appears to be a need to establish better communication, compatible objectives, equality of partnership and of joint decision-making in terms of establishing the initial agenda (Nocon 1993). None of these are seen to have been adequately addressed by the health of the nation strategy, yet recognition of the importance of the principle of collaboration for establishing a policy for health promotion is surely of paramount importance.

The White Paper as a health promotion initiative

In conclusion, therefore, it may be said that the Government's *The Health of the Nation* White Paper has represented an important step towards establishing a change in health policy. *The Health of the Nation* was not the first policy document which laid down a strategy for health outside of the WHO.[1] It does indeed owe much to the ideas for the future of global health care to this organisation and much of the policy contained in the White Paper is a direct result of the work of the WHO. This said, however, the health of the nation strategy falls short of offering a real prospect of health promotion for a number of reasons. There are limitations in the scope and number of the selected key areas and it is questionable whether they are challenging enough. There is a possibility that they have been selected because of their ease of attainment and hence the exclusion of areas such as the elderly. The targets set within the key areas have also been criticised for not being based on scientific data and figures appear to have been arrived at eclectically.

Other problems with the health of the nation in terms of health promotion concerns its failure to offer definitions of health, ill-health, illness and disability. Yet these words provide the very bases on which the document is grounded and in failing to establish what they actually mean, it is difficult to understand what is meant by improvements or changes in them. The ideas behind health promotion offer a complex and multidisciplinary approach to health problems, but *The Health of the Nation* has only really offered a dilution of these ideas. It oversimplifies the causes of illness and exaggerates the importance of lifestyle and its effects on health outcomes. There is also a real failure to attempt to understand the causes of health, therefore rendering the policy limited to disease prevention as opposed to true health promotion.

Finally, there is much talk of variation in health or inequalities in the availability and access to healthcare in the White Paper, while there is no mention whatsoever of the need to establish policies which tackle the real problems of poverty, homelessness and unemployment. Without this it is difficult to accept that the strategy could have any real impact on the health of the nation.

Note

1   That honour belongs to Finland, who brought theirs in 1985.

7

SEXUAL HEALTH PROMOTION AND ITS EVALUATION

Health promotion and HIV/AIDS

With the increase of sexually transmitted diseases and the advent of HIV, sexual health promotion is an important discipline. Since the British Government's publication on *The Health of the Nation* (see Chapter 6), which identifies sexual health as one of its key areas for improving the health of the population, there has been a move away from the term 'HIV prevention' to 'sexual health promotion' in an attempt to incorporate such wider prevention activities as reproductive health and sexually transmitted diseases as well as HIV infection (Alcorn 1996). For the purpose of this chapter, the author will focus on sexual, rather than reproductive, health and look more closely at the social and behavioural aspects of sexual health promotion, rather than at the costs and benefits of medical treatments.

In this, particular attention has been paid to HIV and AIDS and this is used to illustrate some of the problems inherent in sexual health promotion, such as risk behaviour and the relationship between knowledge and beliefs. In such an assessment of the effectiveness of sexual health promotion, the author highlights the difficulties in measuring health behaviour change. First, it is important to lay the foundation to this discussion by defining terms used and then to give an overview of models and approaches used in sexual health promotion.

Any work relating to the promotion of sexual health has to recognise the diversity of human sexual behaviour and the differing views on sexuality and finally on what constitutes sexual health promotion. Sexuality itself is hard to define and it is much more complex than suggested by its purely biological function. 'Sexuality is more a question of identity and links closely to a person's sense of self' (Aggleton and Tyrer 1994). Sexual expression varies enormously and it has long been known that there are no links between sex or gender or sexuality, so it is from this starting point that sexual health promotion must begin.

70

Determining the discourse

So what is sexual health? The Terrence Higgins Trust (cited by Aggleton and Tyrer 1994) recognise that sexual health includes 'physical and emotional well-being, as well as the avoidance of sexually transmitted diseases and unwanted pregnancies, with an overall focus on the practice of safer sex'. George (cited by Alcorn 1996) writes 'sexual health describes the effects that sexuality can have upon health and that health can have upon sexuality'. The WHO concluded in 1987 (cited by Aggleton and Tyrer 1994) that 'due to the range of individual, cultural and social differences and the various patterns of lifestyle, social and gender roles, there can be no single definition of a sexually healthy individual'.

Sexual health promotion, therefore, has been defined in a variety of broad terms because, like health and illness themselves, definitions cannot be specific because the terms are subjective and relative. French and George (cited by Alcorn 1996) view sexual health promotion 'as an umbrella term to describe any intervention which aims to: promote sexual well-being; prevent HIV, other STD's and unwanted pregnancies'. Likewise Curtis writes:

> When one considers that HIV is only the most serious of a range of sexually transmissible agents, including several viruses which are as yet incurable, and that even curable infections such as gonorrhoea, chlamydis and syphilis continue to take their toll of pain, infertility and human misery, it is apparent that the significance of sexual behaviour for public health extends well beyond the prevention of AIDS, and that purely treatment-orientated approaches hold no solution to the problem.
>
> (cited by Alcorn 1996)

There is now a definition for HIV/AIDS health promotion which the WHO created to cover the activities required to contain the spread of HIV: 'as the culture-specific process which seeks to influence positively the relevant health practices of individuals and groups so as to prevent the transmission of HIV infection' (cited in Pye 1990).

Do preventive strategies empower?

In the early 1980s HIV prevention strategies were built on the preventive and educational models which were based on coercion and blame, rather than on support and empowerment. The first media campaigns used imagery, such as tombstones and references to plague, to frighten people into acquiescence. This caused people to either over- or under-react. The lessons learnt were that proposed behavioural changes have to be attractive and individuals must believe that they are personally at risk. Indeed, individuals must feel that they can both achieve behaviour change at an acceptable cost and that behaviour change will avoid HIV infection. Telling people the facts, and then assuming that this will lead to automatic behaviour change, has proven to be relatively ineffective in sexual health education.

Likewise, the early prevention strategies had faults. They were biased towards making people 'differentiably' responsible for their behaviour by implying social disapproval of certain lifestyles, which apportioned blame to certain groups in society. Instead of stopping the spread of HIV, policy-makers and the media alike seemed determined to stop certain activities and preferences, such as homosexuality, promiscuity, prostitution, drug use and so on. To counter this sort of thing, education about sexual health must involve far more than the provision of fact and information.

It is now recognised that self-empowerment and community-based initiatives constitute the most effective intervention (Aggleton and Moody 1992; McEwan and Bhopal 1991). The self-empowerment model is favoured because it extends the educational approach by giving individuals choice and power, and the collective approach is preferable because campaigns need to be seen to be at a grass roots level so that people have the choice about how best to realise their local population agendas and to target needs. It is argued by many that social change should ideally come from the bottom up rather than the top down and that it succeeds through the involvement of the community, those threatened and concerned and those whose every day life is affected (McEwan and Bhopal 1991; Kickbusch 1994; Aggleton and Moody 1992; Tones 1981). Aggleton and Tyrer (1994) take this further and argue that 'for education about sexual health to be most effective, it is important to attempt to develop and promote an awareness of wider issues such as oppression, gender inequality, distribution of power and cultural expressions'.

Sexual health promotion can take place in a number of different settings, for example, in general practice, family planning services and in genito-urinary clinics (GU). In the UK, the number of cases seen in GU clinics has doubled over the past fifteen years and now amount to nearly 740,000 new cases a year (Adler 1995). The reason for this is multifactorial. For example, the introduction of the pill and other non-protective barrier methods of contraception is a factor. However, Adler also argues that improved service provision and contact tracing may also be responsible for the increased numbers presenting to GU clinics, so it is difficult to make assumptions about numbers in real terms.

The aim of sexual health promotion in GU clinics is to 'offer prompt diagnosis and treatment, minimise the incidence of complications, trace and treat the infected partners of patients and educate patients, the public, and health care workers' (Adler 1995). Early diagnosis and treatment for many sexually transmitted diseases is not only cheap but also effective in controlling the spread of such diseases. Methods of control are through epidemiological treatment, which can help to reduce the infection 'pool' in the community; raising awareness through education and protecting the health of individuals who are unaware of gonococcal, chlamydial or syphilis infection through contact tracing. The prevention of costly long-term disability is of crucial importance. For example, most cases of pelvic inflammatory disease are preventable. The problem is caused by a sexually transmitted disease, which, when left untreated, will lead to long-term damage and suffering in women and this, in turn, means long-term support and a drain on medical resources. Evidence suggests that early diagnosis and prevention is the only effective way to manage this difficult condition (Adler 1995; Mann *et al.* 1996).

Social/psychological constraints

However, there are many problems associated with encouraging people to participate in the promotion of their sexual health. For example, there are practical problems such as access to services. Although there are 240 departments of GU medicine in the UK, there is still a tendency for these services to be located in dingy basements or down dark alley-ways. Facilities, surely, should alleviate, not create, stigma and be readily accessible for self-referral (Adler 1995; McHaffie 1993). Other problems for people attending clinics are embarrassment, fear, and confidentiality. 'Some departments are named after physicians, apostles or battles and others are termed "special departments" or given a number or letter' (Adler 1995). This can also confuse and alienate people when accessing a clinic.

There are also particular problems in the provision of healthcare for women in that the services are split between primary care, the gynaecologist, GU services and family planning. Thus, without integrated facilities contacting and treating sexual partners, and without collaboration between specialities, this can be problematic or inefficient (Mann *et al.* 1996). The law can also inhibit access to support/healthcare services with its legislation on the age of consent. For those under-age women or young gay men, who may be particularly vulnerable to infection, reaching this population to access and promote sexual health is made even more difficult.

It is the issue of HIV/AIDS, which, more than any other factor, has forced society to address the areas of sex and sexuality in all its forms. *The Health of the Nation* has described HIV and AIDS as 'the greatest new threat to public health this century' (DOH 1992). In the Government's White Paper on *The Health of the Nation* (DOH 1992), one of the five key areas identified for change is sexual health because of the rapid spread of HIV/AIDS. The objectives are to reduce the incidence of HIV infection and other STDs by strengthening monitoring and surveillance and by providing services for the effective diagnosis and treatment of these infections. The target is to reduce:

the national incidence of gonorrhoea by at least 20 per cent by 1995;
the proportion of drug users who report needle sharing from a fifth in
1990 to no more than a tenth in 1997;
by at least half the rate of conceptions among the under 16s by the year
2000.

Whether this is achievable will be discussed later. Firstly, though, it is
important to consider some of the fundamental dilemmas associated with
the issues of HIV/AIDS. As Weeks pointed out (cited by Scott and Freeman
1995) 'what gives AIDS a particular power is its ability to represent a host of
fears, anxieties and problems in our current, post-permissive society'. As
Scott and Freeman (1995) argue, these risks and problems are managed
in different 'social arenas', namely in public policy, by medicine and by
individuals.

Public health is orientated to controlling disease in such a way as for it
to permit 'surveillance' of 'sources of infection'. In the case of HIV, unlike
other infectious diseases,

> the usefulness of surveillance as a method of evaluation effectiveness
> is seriously limited by the particularities of infection with HIV, such
> as the stigma attached, the long latency period, the dynamic of the
> epidemic and the absence of a vaccine or an effective treatment.
>
> (Friedrich *et al*. 1994)

So the question arises should authoritarian approaches be enforced to
minimise the spread of the disease? Consider, for example, the criminalisation
of a West Midlands man accused of deliberately infecting four women with
the virus and discussed by government ministers in 1992 (*Guardian* 1992 cited
by Scott and Freeman 1995), or the liberal approach of prevention by
identifying the individual's behaviour and looking to change this through the
provision of information, education, advice and support. A strategy put
forward for the 1990s about the nation's health states that, 'Human behaviour
does not reflect individual choices alone so much as the powerful influence of
the social, economic and political environments that lie substantially beyond
the control of the individuals who are affected by them'. This recognised that
the state of the nation's public health cannot rest on the responsibility of
individuals alone. There must also be government action; the two must
interact and need to work hand in hand (Smith and Jacobson 1988).

Medicalisation versus health promotion

Modern medicine has had little impact on the spread of HIV as it has not
been able to find a cure or vaccine and is unlikely to for some years to come
(Scott and Freeman 1995; Holland and Fullerton 1995). Medicine can define

areas of risk and prevention but cannot remove them. 'Even where effective therapies do exist, for example against syphilis and gonorrhoea, their spread cannot be successfully contained by medical therapies alone' (Holland and Fullerton 1995). Understanding risk-taking behaviour and preventing the spread of these diseases has called into play many other factors, such as contact tracing and raising awareness.

'Since diseases that are prevented are necessarily unreported, the success of a preventative procedure is more difficult to demonstrate than that of a therapy' (Smith and Jacobson 1988). It is difficult to prove that those who remain healthy have done so because of a prevention programme. It is also argued that prevention seems less efficient than treatment, because money is being directed towards a healthy population and that outcome is not necessarily tangible or immediate, unlike the medication for someone who is sick (Smith and Jacobson 1988). 'The focus of health education has shifted from disease process to personal behaviour, as evidenced by the dominance of "lifestyle" in discussions of prevention' (Scott and Freeman 1995). However, health promotion within the context of the health service is still dominated by the biomedical model which is criticised for being narrow and too medicalised (Scott 1992).

Principal health education messages have been to promote safer sex, the core elements of which are negotiation and condom use.

> Safer sex is premised on an awareness and acceptance of risk and, in turn, on the production of trust. In this context, trust may be understood as the solution to a specific problem of risk. In turn, this raises the question of the relationship between risk-awareness and risk-avoidance.
>
> (Scott and Freeman 1995)

Individuals have to assess their own risk as it is impossible to arbitrarily assume that high risks of HIV infection attach to certain individuals. Health promotion can assist in this dialogue, but negotiation in any relationship can never be complete or absolute because it is dependent on so many hidden factors. 'One of the reasons why it is so difficult to translate anxiety about HIV and AIDS into rational dialogue is precisely because it calls trust and intimacy, the insecure bases of fragile sexual identities, into question' (Scott and Freeman 1995).

Trust, intimacy and personal autonomy

Trust, therefore, may be viewed as a solution to the prevention of the transmission of HIV infection within relationships but the problems here are that for many young women, for example, 'the need to trust has its roots in romantic, feminine discourse and is likely to result in an understanding of love as prophylactic' (Scott and Freeman 1995). Trust is seen not only in terms of trusting a partner, but in people's perception of risk. For example, 'It won't happen to me', 'I'm clean', 'I'm straight'. 'Trust is neither in a relationship nor in a rational process of risk assessment, but in the cultural understandings of sexuality and in gendered sexual scripts' (Scott and Freeman 1995).

Holland *et al.* (1992) explain in their study of the negotiation of safer sex, that for young women this is problematic because of their subordinate role and this can contribute to unsafe sexual behaviour, regardless of the dangers.

> The understanding of sexual risk-taking by young women, and the promotion of safer sex for young heterosexuals, will depend on the extent to which we can make connections between the sexual pleasures and their personal empowerment in managing their own lives.
>
> (Holland *et al.* 1992)

Promoting sexual health, therefore, is a complex dialogue between health promoter and the client and the ability of both to put those health education messages into practice.

Central to much HIV prevention work is the dynamic of power, not only for women but for everyone alike. Aggleton describes this as

> the power that denies women the opportunity to participate fully in sexual decision-making; the power that limits the freedom of lesbians and gay men to express their sexuality openly and without fear of attack; the power that denies those who are physically or intellectually disabled the right to a fulfilling sex life; the power that denies young people access to the information they may need to protect themselves against unwanted pregnancy and STD; and the power that encourages an understanding of black people's sexuality as being different from and inferior to that of whites.
>
> (Aggleton and Moody 1992)

It is important to understand these underlying issues when discussing sexual health promotion because any assessment of its effectiveness would have to recognise relative levels of empowerment (or its reverse) in the context of marginalisation of various types.

Perception of risk

Fundamental to the hypothesis of health promotion is the expectation that it alters people's perception of risk. 'Successful HIV intervention campaigns would need to address the situations in which risk behaviour occurs and, not least, the power relations which limit or eliminate health choices' (Bloor

1995). The psychological context assumes immense importance. For example, when individuals are faced with dealing directly with a problem they often go into 'denial (the problem does not exist), displacement (the problem has nothing to do with me) and delay (I'll change my behaviour one day, but not right now)' (Aggleton and Tyrer 1994). There are many theories that are put forward to explain the variations in individuals' perceptions of risk. The 'health belief model' is most widely used to describe HIV-related risk behaviour (Bloor 1995). For example, the health belief model views health behaviour in association with interlinked perceptions:

> Firstly, the individual must perceive him/herself as vulnerable or susceptible to a health threat, such as HIV infection. Secondly that health threat has to be perceived as having serious consequences. Thirdly, the protective action that is potentially available to avoid that health threat has to be perceived as an effective safeguard. And fourthly, taking the protective action has to be perceived to have benefits which outweigh the perceived costs.
>
> (Bloor 1995)

However, issues which must be considered are power dynamics within a relationship (for example, the negotiation of safer sex), constraint verses choice, immediate incentives of risk taking, etc. Sharing needles, for example, may outweigh the thought of the long-term risk.

Some would argue that the health belief model does not work because 'there is inconsistent evidence that knowledge of risk is related to behaviour change' (Cohen and Chwalow 1995). It is all too obvious that individuals often have a poor ability to perceive risk because people find it hard to recognise their own susceptibility. It could be said that health behaviour is the wrong domain and that many people have more immediate needs that outweigh the outcome of unprotected sex and they may be prepared to take risks accordingly. Knowledge, attitudes and beliefs are as much a consequence of behaviour as the cause of behaviour – basically they all measure the same thing. Information can result in dramatically different behaviours given different environments or times, for information is not static and a focus on the individual behaviour, for pressure from others can shape behaviour. With all this in mind the question now remains: Does sexual heath promotion work? Given the complexities and dynamics briefly outlined above, it is hard to prove, as shall now be explained.

The problem of assessment

There are a variety of processes by which the quality of HIV/AIDS health education and health promotion programmes are assessed. It is necessary to briefly explain the difference between monitoring and evaluation and to explain some of the key issues and techniques that are commonly used.

The WHO have defined monitoring as: 'the process of collecting and analysing information about the implementation of the programme: it involves regular checking to see whether programme activities are being carried out as planned so that problems can be discerned and dealt with' (WHO 1986).

Evaluation is described as:

the process of collecting and analysing information about the effectiveness and impact of either particular phases of the programme or the programme as a whole. Evaluation also involves assessing programme achievements for the purpose of detecting and solving problems and planning for the future.

(WHO 1986)

Monitoring, therefore, is concerned more closely with the ongoing implementation of a programme, whereas evaluation is concerned with the programme's effectiveness. There are two types of evaluation frequently used in HIV/AIDS health education programmes – outcome and process evaluation.

There are many components to outcome evaluation but its principal aim is to measure changes that are cognitive (e.g. knowledge about HIV and its modes of transmission), attitudinal (e.g. views about people with HIV/AIDS) and behavioural (e.g. changes in person or group behaviour) (Aggleton and Moody 1992). Alternatively, the outcome measures can be to estimate the number of people reached by a particular initiative or the amount of resources used (Aggleton and Moody 1992). In all cases goals (statements of intent), objectives (desired end result) and performance targets (intermediate results), must be made so reliable that valid indicators (data on changes that have taken place) can be achieved.

Process evaluation examines how and why the outcomes in the latter were achieved. It is more qualitative and descriptive rather than quantifiable. 'The emphasis in process evaluation therefore is on studying the process of learning that takes place through health education and health promotion and on identifying factors that facilitate or impede individual and group behaviour change' (Aggleton and Moody 1992). It looks at the how and why questions, that is, it explores different perspectives of the empowerment and community action approaches and incorporates the overall picture of management, workers as well as clients (Scott 1992).

It is important to evaluate, not only to assess the effectiveness of any given campaign, but also to monitor progress; to measure impact; to maximise cost-efficiency; to share experience. Ultimately it is an essential planning tool. However, the HIV/AIDS field is a particularly sensitive one and data can often be manipulated or misinterpreted because it is a political as well as a social problem and one that highlights moral and ethical issues. By its nature 'evaluation is never a neutral and objective activity' (Aggleton and Moody 1992). Thus particular attention must be given to the reasons for evaluation and the selection of methodology.

Very often the target setting for HIV/AIDS is given to those problems which are measurable but, as Johnson argues (1991), setting targets for risk reduction and monitoring long-term risk behaviour is required. However, it is hard to measure outcome and behaviour change. It depends on what is being measured and for whom and any health-related behaviour cannot be seen in isolation from the individual's situation and circumstances.

> It is a mistake to focus on outcomes as separate entities for, unless an understanding is developed of the context in which health promotion takes place and the processes through which this work is carried out, even if seemingly positive outcomes are identified, there may be no means of explaining how they arose or how they can be reproduced
>
> (Scott 1992)

Holland and Fullerton (1995) state that many evaluations make claims about the effects of interventions but this does little to establish effectiveness. They undertook a study to assess the effectiveness of 886 HIV/AIDS health promotion and education interventions. There were 114 reports of evaluations and these were studied by the authors for effectiveness and sound methodology. Five (33 per cent) of the methodologically sound studies were judged effective by authors and three (20 per cent) by reviewers. Authors judged 33 per cent of the flawed studies effective compared to 9 per cent for reviewers. The largest difference between authors and reviewers for the flawed studies was that 43 per cent were considered unclear by reviewers because of methodological problems and/or lack of necessary information. Overall, there was 54 per cent agreement between authors and reviewers on effectiveness and in 6 per cent of cases some agreement as to some effect; in 16 per cent of cases authors said the intervention was effective and the reviewers disagreed, and in 21 per cent of cases the reviewers judged the intervention to be unclear or ineffective when the authors' view was that it was partially effective.

According to Holland and Fullerton (1995), randomised control trials (RCTs) are the only effective and reliable way of establishing effectiveness of different types of intervention. Comparing the pre- and post-intervention measures against themselves, rather than a control population, provides inadequate data. They argue that 'it is the very complexity and multiplicity of factors influencing health attitudes and behaviours that strengthens the case for properly designed RCTs'. RCTs have been favoured by the medical profession in situations where there is uncertainty about whether a treatment or programme works. However, the urgency of the AIDS epidemic and the moral and ethical issues involved have meant that the 'lack of time justified lack of evaluation, and the "unethics" of withholding from anyone something that might work functioned to dilute even further the goal of establishing effective ways of tackling the progress or spread of the disease' (Holland and Fullerton 1995).

Outcome measures therefore have been limited because of the lack of evidence that could have been supplied by the RCTs. This, coupled with the pressure from management for interventions to supply information relevant to particular audits and the gap between research and policy and the inappropriate decisions made by policy-makers, despite the findings of sound policies, have led to major obstacles in limiting the spread of HIV and AIDS. It is not just the prevention initiatives that need to be looked at for effectiveness in promoting sexual health, but also the context in which they are being provided. Very often there is a conflict between prevention and cure; management and funding and evaluation are often used as the tools with which to battle this out (Scott 1992).

Evaluation needs to be seen in the context of a whole range of aspects. It must reflect a consideration of: the individual, future funding, ongoing support mechanisms for client, workers and agencies, as well as being a tool to measure effectiveness. As Holland and Fullerton demonstrate, problems that have arisen within the field of HIV/AIDS health promotion have been through design fault (choice of methodology), lack of consensus about the choice of appropriate outcome measures, e.g. the biological outcomes; behavioural outcome; reduction of risk behaviours; protective behaviours; psychological outcomes. Added to this is the complication of measuring outcomes when the HIV incubation period is so long.

From the variety of evaluation outcomes measures mentioned, it is easy to see how multidisciplinary the field of HIV/AIDS is. Therefore, the variety of ideologies and understandings attending the professional discipline (medical, psychological, management) are also great. The goals are shared but there are many differing angles, such as, 'to improve local people's knowledge of HIV/AIDS' or 'to reduce the spread of HIV infection in the local population' (Scott 1992). Is the prevention programme to assess the potential saving of life, raising awareness in the whole population or in a certain sub-group in the prevention of the spread of HIV or in reducing discrimination by changing society's attitudes, which in turn could improve people's quality of life and enable them to function within the community (Godfrey and Tolley 1992)? Measuring quantity of life (number of life years) and quality of life is itself subjective.

Health promotion, in terms of HIV/AIDS, is sometimes evaluated in terms of behaviour change. More often than not this is what is required by the funders. The US Panel on the Evaluation of AIDS Interventions recommended behavioural measures as the primary outcome for most AIDS intervention programmes (Coyle cited by Holland and Fullerton 1995) as seroconversion rates are too problematic to measure because of the length of incubation and the use of this outcome measure requires large sample sizes. As Holland and Fullerton (1995) point out 'a trial taking HIV infection as the outcome measure and using favourable assumptions (50% decrease in new infections due to the programme, 5% baseline seroconversion rate and 70% follow-up rate would require recruitment of over 2,500 injecting drug users (School of Public Health and Institute for Health Policy Studies 93)) would be immensely difficult to mount'. They also argue that 'the use of behavioural measures as "proxy" indicators of the likelihood of infection requires a sound understanding, based on careful prior mapping of the relationships between individual behaviours and the chances of acquiring HIV'. Scott (1992) argues that the relationship between knowledge, beliefs and behaviour is weak and, therefore, using behaviour change as the central activity on which to focus HIV, renders the value of health promotion limited.

It is simply unrealistic to develop a yardstick for behaviour in the context of HIV/AIDS and then use it to assess everyone's progress . . . . We must learn not to use common-sense categories and labels to tidy up the messiness and variety of everyday life.

(Scott 1992)

Critique of evaluation

Health promotion has been under the spotlight to reduce and control the spread of HIV. Pressure is being put on health workers to get quantifiable empirical evidence to assess the effectiveness of HIV prevention but, because HIV is a complex social issue as well as a disease, outcome-focused and goal-orientated evaluation in this context often raises more questions of uncertainty, because it does not constitute a purely scientific problem. A good example is condom use and safer sex. This has been central to many health education campaigns and measured according to the uptake of condom-related behaviour.

However, as seen by the data produced by Holland et al. (1992), condom use is linked to meanings and understandings which cannot easily be measured and to the existence of male control (Scott 1992). Outcome measures that record the number of times condoms are used cannot guarantee condom use in the future or the complexities of negotiating their use. It is these hidden influences which need to be analysed and understood in order to promote effective HIV/AIDS health promotion (Scott 1992). 'Poor measurement is worse than no measurement and, rather than being exact and scientific, a focus on outcome alone is likely to produce shallow results based on inadequate and superficial analysis' (Scott 1992).

The need for secure resources and the competition for funds between the fields of prevention, treatment and research makes evaluation particularly important, especially as estimates of HIV infection have been lower than predicted (Godfrey and Tolley 1992). 'Early projections of HIV infection rates overestimated the numbers of AIDS cases in Britain, largely because behaviour change among gay men had led to fewer cases than expected' (McEwan and Bhopal 1991).

However, predictions are difficult to make and for these to be useful, data on sexual behaviour of the population at risk, changes in sexual behaviour over time and the relationship between HIV infection and disease and the length of time it takes to develop AIDS, are needed (Smith and Jacobson 1988; Wellings et al. 1994).

> Efforts to mount effective public health education campaigns, to predict the likely extent and pattern of the spread of HIV, and to plan services for those effected have all been hampered by the absence of reliable data on sexual behaviour.
>
> (Wellings et al. 1994)

The aim of the 'Sexual Behaviour in Britain Study', carried out by the National Survey of Sexual Attitudes and Lifestyles, was to provide data that would increase the understanding of the transmission patterns of HIV and assist in the selection of appropriate and effective health education strategies for epidemic control. They argue that preventive intervention needs an understanding of patterns of human sexuality in order to design effective interventions and advice on risk reduction (Wellings et al. 1994). This is backed up by Johnson (1991) who argues that targets for HIV and AIDS have floundered largely on the problems of assessing the rate of spread of HIV in Britain. This is a result of both limited epidemological data and lack of baseline population estimates of risk behaviour necessary to define the size of behaviour change required to control the epidemic.

The problem of risk behaviour and of understanding how to modify such action is central to the prevention and control of HIV/AIDS. However, as discussed, finding an outcome measure to assess the effectiveness of such initiatives is difficult when one examines health behaviour and the complex issues that make behaviour change problematic and then add to this the difficulty of attributing changes to a particular education programme. The effectiveness of sexual health promotion is, therefore, very difficult to assess, because of the lack of data and of concrete evidence to back up such claims. However, the challenge of HIV/AIDS has clarified many weaknesses, imbalances and inconsistencies in past health promotion efforts. The WHO projects that the decade of the 1990s will provide greater pressures, expectations and opportunities for HIV/AIDS health promotion to take place. Despite the conflict and lack of consensus regarding the meaning and intended outcomes of sexual health initiatives, this should not preclude or diminish the importance and significance that health promotion can play in the prevention of HIV/AIDS.

8

DIET AND HEALTH
PROMOTION

Empowerment, intrusion and ethics

All lifestyle issues embody tremendous paradoxes for the health promoter. Consider smoking, for instance. The negative health consequences of smoking are now widely known. Does government action on advertising not intrude on people's freedom under the law to make a living in advertising, and does not such interference constitute also a violation of the right to choose (whether to be healthy or not) on the part of the people who might want to look at a cigarette advertisement? Some of these ethical issues will be considered in Chapter 9. But at least the smoking issue is reasonably simple. Whereas a drinking lifestyle is shrouded in ambiguity by statistical and epidemiological debate about how much liquor (and what type) is good for one or, more to the point, past what amount per week does it become harmful, that is not true of tobacco use. Any amount of tobacco smoking is deleterious to one's health and even to the health of other people in the vicinity.

The situation becomes even more thorny if we consider diet. Eating is not only a primary function, but is invested for almost everyone with deep psychological social and even spiritual meaning. Very few things are as intimate and personal as what one chooses to eat. Although the physiology of food intake is hugely complex, rendering nutrition a minefield of ambiguity and past scientific errors, we now have generated a respectable body of reliable information about much of it. The slogan: 'you are what you eat' has exercised a wide influence and people are increasingly becoming diet-conscious and interest among lay people about practical nutrition is spreading. This certainly has opened up opportunities for health education about nutrition. What about health promotion?

What food we eat

Generally considered a prerequisite to a healthy existence is a balanced and nutritious diet. If our food intake lacks essential nutrients, is poorly balanced nutritionally, or includes harmful agents, our health will eventually

84

suffer. Becoming prone to nutritional deficiency diseases and increasing our likelihood of developing diseases such as diabetes, coronary artery diseases and certain cancers (e.g. Robbins 1991; Lobstein 1991) are inextricably related.

In what ways can dietary health be promoted? This chapter will consider that question, with particular reference to adults, and focusing mainly on foodstuffs rather than fluids. With children the issue is not less important, but much less ethically ambiguous. There is no real problem in telling one's children what to eat, even though it is bedevilled by logistic and psychological problems. But a major problem for health promotion is adult eating lifestyles and how they might be modified.

Although the nutritional status of the British population has improved immensely over the past century, there are still many concerns. In part, these are related to the numerous and continuing changes to the food-chain as well as to the meteoric rise of food advertising by manufacturers and retailers. These concerns are also related to poverty as well as to lack of consumer empowerment, especially among certain parts of the population.

Changes to the British diet over time

Prior to the advent of rail transportation and the intervention of canning and refrigeration, the British people generally ate locally grown or raised foodstuffs, including vegetables and fruit in their season. If certain nutrients or trace elements were lacking, nutritional deficiency diseases would result, often very locally. Goitre, or 'Derbyshire neck', in parts of the Pennines from a lack of iodine is an outstanding example. Britain had moved from being an agrarian society to an industrialised one by the middle of the nineteenth century. However, industrialisation itself frequently brought poverty and gross malnutrition, including rickets, to those who lived in the often appalling overcrowded and squalid housing conditions of the industrial cities of Victorian Britain.

When recruitment for the Boer War highlighted large numbers of men unfit to fight, the British Government acknowledged the poor health status of many of the British people and, thereafter, the emergent science of nutrition was applied increasingly to feeding the nation. As a result, Britain quickly became a world leader in understanding these issues. Regrettably, these insights tended to remain largely academic, only affecting practice significantly in times of war. Thus, during the Second World War, for example, food rationing and fortification of certain foods was introduced (Drummond et al. 1957), and these changes led to an improvement in the health of the British population, especially improvements in infant and maternal mortality (Blight and Scanlon 1986). In more recent times the composition of the British population has become increasingly multicultural and there have been marked changes in eating lifestyles countrywide. 'Fast' and convenience foods have also become more a part of the nation's diet.

Consumer choice

We can justifiably claim in Britain that today food is plentiful, varied and readily available at local markets, shopping malls, large supermarket chains, corner shops, restaurants and 'take-aways'. Although much more is known now about dietary requirements and nutritional values by both the general public and the relevant professionals, the challenge for today's consumer is how to shop wisely for food. We live in a world in which biotechnology (applied to animals and foodstuffs) is a reality (Donnellan 1996a), and in which some foods contain little of the ingredients we expect. Indeed, it is not unusual for some food products to be little more than a chemical *mélange* of artificial flavourings, preservatives and colourings. Food and agricultural scientists continue to discover ways to alter crops so that they can be grown more rapidly and more economically, and to rear animals as quickly as possible, often keeping them in overcrowded and unhealthy conditions.

Currently careful and detailed market research invariably precedes the launching of new food products (Advertising Association 1984). Food manufacturers and retailers spend vast sums of money to advertise on billboards, television and cinema, and in magazines and newspapers, sometimes with the intent to entice us into buying highly processed foods of poor nutritional value, 'empty calories' from saturated fats and/or highly processed sugars (Advertising Association 1984; Cannon 1987). 'Junk' foods are frequently advertised on television at peak viewing times for children, thus undermining parental authority on diet (Donnellan 1996b).

In such a commercial environment, it is natural that economics, and indeed politics, have great sway over decisions regarding the food we eat. The food industry, which is controlled by a small number of 'giant' organisations such as Unilever, has become large and extremely powerful. Challenging these powerful organisations are various food lobbyists, such as Lobstein (1993) and Walker and Cannon (1985). How assured can the British public be when they are eating foods which will endanger health, when pesticide residues, for instance, are known to remain in some foods, when many livestock receive antibiotics and growth hormones, and when foods are frequently irradiated (Taylor and Taylor 1990)? We have recently seen the bovine spongiform encephalopathy (BSE) crisis (e.g., Arthur 1996; *Which?* 1996), an increasing number of food poisoning outbreaks (e.g., *Which?* 1995; *Daily Mail* 1996), as well as the increasing production of genetically modified foods (e.g., Brown 1996; Clover 1996) have received national media coverage and evoked deep public concern (Campbell 1990).

While the food we eat in the 1990s is much more varied, much of it is also more highly processed than was the case even thirty years ago.

Need the British diet be a health promotion issue?

Evidently, there have been vast changes to the British diet during the past centuries. Severe malnutrition and starvation are now rarities, and more people are living longer than they did a century ago. As in several other European countries (Usher 1996), the British people are growing taller. In view of all this, is there then a need for large financial expenditure and concerted efforts to be directed towards health promotion activities relating to the British diet? Does the current state of public health warrant it, and, if so, how can health promoters seek to bring about change?

A decade ago, Cannon, a journalist with an interest in food and health, looked closely at research findings and the opinions of eminent people in government, science, medicine and industry. His conclusion was that the British diet was among the unhealthiest in Europe (Cannon 1987). For instance, in 1985, survey findings were published on the dietary habits of 15- to 25-year-olds, many of whom were found to have lower than the recommended level of folic acid, an important indicator as to whether certain fresh vegetables were being eaten. Women aged 19 to 21 years were found to have intakes of 116 micrograms of folic acid a day, considerably lower than the UK (Ministry of Agriculture, Fisheries and Food (MAFF)) recommended levels of 300 micrograms per day (Bull 1985 referred to in Cannon 1987). This age group included women planning to conceive, and who, without dietary supplements, would suffer nutritional deficiencies which could harm their unborn child.

Cannon (1987) also addresses other dietary issues, including increased sugar intake (linked to the increased likelihood of diabetes, heart disease and dental decay) and consumption of additives (what the public as well as food manufacturers do and do not know about them). Principally, he is concerned about the Government's lack of openness regarding the state of public ill-health as well as about certain research reports. Reports which shed a less favourable light have even been held back or discreetly published without the usual fanfare of publicity (e.g., the National Advisory Council on Nutrition Education's report in 1983; see Potrykus 1989; Townsend and Davidson 1982). The power of the food industry, as well as of Members of Parliament often seeming more concerned about vote-winning issues than the health, or ill-health, of the nation, is an ongoing concern of Cannon.

Then, also in the 1980s, Catford and Ford (1984) compared the 'state of the public ill health' in the UK with that of most other countries in the then European Economic Community and Scandinavia. Commenting that the mortality among men and women aged 45–64 years (an age when people are usually economically productive and have younger and older dependants of their family to care for) was considerable higher in the UK than elsewhere, they suggested that unhealthy lifestyles, including poor nutrition, probably provided part of the answer. Cardiovascular disease was noted as being an important cause of premature death among this age group.

Government response

While Cannon and others (e.g., *Lancet* 1986) were deeply concerned that the Government did not readily accept findings which highlighted the unhealthy nature of the British diet, other writers, notably Anderson (1986; also Le Fanu 1986), considered findings which Cannon and others draw upon as being poorly substantiated. Marks (1991) commented that the quality of food available to the general public had never been higher. As well, without modern agricultural methods and industrial handling and processing of food, it would be very difficult to feed the population of cities such as London. Six years after all of this, the White Paper *The Health of the Nation* (DOH 1992) was published. For the first time ever, the Government had identified specific health targets for England similar to those most western nations face. These health challenges all affect diet and include the reduction of inequities, notably those relating to economic status. In Britain, increasing unemployment, growth in the number of single parent families, and increasing numbers of retired people have led to a doubling in the number of people reliant on means-tested benefits, despite a rise in the average household income during the 1980s (George 1993). Epp (1986) identified two other challenges. These are the need to find new and more effective ways to prevent the occurrence of injuries, illnesses, and chronic conditions and their resulting disabilities, and, secondly, the challenge of enhancing people's capacity to cope.

Also included in Epp's framework are three particular challenges which Naegele (1992) describes as: encouraging a social climate that favours public participation, strengthening community health services to become more supportive of personal and community needs, and, thirdly, co-ordinating public policy and incorporating health as a consideration into the policy agendas of all sectors.

When it is considered that the adequate intake of nutrients is a basic human requirement, and that sound nutrition is recognised as an important factor in the prevention of various illnesses, in the maintenance of a sound constitution, and in the development of our intellectual capacity (Brown and Pollitt 1996), dietary health appears to be worthy of promotion, both as an entity on its own and in conjunction with other health promotion incentives. Therefore, it is no accident that dietary health promotion is now widely considered to be within Epp's identified mechanisms. Though each mechanism will be considered separately, health promotion efforts do not necessarily utilise one mechanism alone.

Focus 1: self-care

Self-care is envisaged as encompassing decisions and actions individuals take in the interest of their own health. While there is considerable support for individuals to increase their nutritional awareness, for instance among those who promote the notion of 'wellness' (e.g., Ardell 1977), how easy, in fact, is it for the general public to decide if foods are truly nutritious and safe to eat? Can the average person really decide if labelling is adequate, if the 'E' numbers (for additives) and various chemical ingredients in foods have relevance to their own and their family's health, and if certain foods are likely to cause infection if they are not cooked in a certain manner? Can we realistically expect the individual to shoulder so much responsibility?

How food preferences are established

It is well understood that provision of dietary information alone is unlikely to change people's nutritional habits. Food preferences and behaviour are learnt from childhood onwards and become an integral part of how we identify ourselves as socio-cultural beings (Lupton 1996). It is interesting to speculate on just how food preferences become established, because they are one of the strongest cultural indicators people have. It is known that very young babies, and this seems to be true in all ethnic groups, are almost entirely tolerant about eating whatever they are fed, unless the food is exceptionally strong tasting. But then, by about the time they are a year old, they suddenly become extremely fastidious, easily accepting some foods but vehemently rejecting others.

To this author, such a state of affairs makes perfectly good sense, in evolutionary and survival terms. When the baby is still too young to walk, crawl or otherwise seek out its own food, it must rely on older people around it to bring food to it. If the people around wished to harm the baby, they could give it unsuitable or poisonous food. But this is only rarely the case. Generally the baby's best survival chances rest with easily accepting what it is given because in all probability the food is given by an adult (usually the mother) with the baby's best interest at heart. However, once the baby can move about on its own, it will constantly be running up against potentially edible items which it can grab and eat without adult intervention. If the baby retained its previous tolerance to taste and texture, it could readily be harmed. But by now it has developed a highly selective sense of taste so that it does not put into its mouth any substance with which it is not already familiar.

In fact, the choice of food we eat is shaped by many factors, including our ethnic heritage (e.g., Helman 1984), our financial status (Driver 1984; Health Education Authority 1989), our religious beliefs (e.g., Mares *et al.* 1985) as well as personal likes and dislikes (Lyman 1989). As previously observed, cultural traditions are often firmly entrenched in childhood and frequently equated with notions of security, stability and love. However, there are an increasing number of people, especially young women, who crave to look like ultra-slim film-stars and models, and these strong desires influence their dietary intake, and their health, as they seek a specific body image (Donnellan 1996b) and to satisfy emotional needs. Bulimia, for instance, has increased three-fold over the past five years (Emmett 1996).

Obviously, if healthy dietary behaviour is to be promoted among individuals, then attitudes and beliefs as well as knowledge become important. The general public can now easily access a large and wide range of dietary information. Written materials, including books and pamphlets, range from general health guides, including everything from nutritional advice to specialised dietary information, such as recommendations for men needing to lose weight (British Heart Foundation 1996), to foods to tempt the terminally ill (Haller 1994). As well, various graphic and easily understood food guides have been developed, which are also appearing in ethnic minority formats (e.g., West London Healthcare NHS Trust 1995). Britain's dinner-plate-shaped food guide (Health Education Authority 1996), Australia's 'healthy diet pyramid' (Open University 1985) and Canada's rainbow-shaped guide (Health and Welfare, Canada 1992) all visually confirm those foods which we should eat more of (cereals, bread, fruit and vegetables) and those we should eat less of (certain fats and sugars) in colour-coded, appropriately-sized sections. In addition, people can also turn to *Which?* magazine or download information from the Internet.

Despite all of this, there is still a place for information and encouragement to be provided in a direct, personal manner, for instance at health promotion market stalls run by health visitors (Brierley *et al.* 1988), and for linking people to specialist groups (e.g., diabetic groups (Kelleher 1994) and Eating Disorder Units). In other words, we are speaking of actually changing a person's cultural responses if we are looking to modify their diet. There are all sorts of psychological implications in this. People will change their behaviour if doing so in a particular manner enhances their sense of social approval and of self-esteem. The two are very closely linked. With respect to food, the British diet has changed radically since the 1960s. In 1964, in Coventry, the author found that cooking with garlic and having wine with the meal were so at variance with the eating culture of his indigenous friends, that many could not enjoy the meals he offered. By the 1970s, with an insurgence of continental influence, 'foreign' food had acquired a certain cachet among the professional classes in Coventry. Even if a British lecturer really did prefer bangers, mash and peas to what was on offer, this was no longer stated. It was felt to reflect on his/her sophistication. Thus, by a combination of the need for social approval and the need to feel good about oneself, dietary habits changed in that group. That meant that it was only a matter of time before it spread more widely. This brings in the question of empowerment and creates a space for health promotion.

Dietary empowerment

Empowering individuals to make healthy dietary choices is obviously an important aspect of health promotion at the 'self-care' level. However, an awareness of the ethical constraints is crucial (Kemm and Close 1995). Although not necessarily prudent, it is the individual's right to be 'unhealthy' (Downie 1983), though 'health' as a concept is differently construed by different people. Providing information that is ethnically and religiously sensitive, taking time to find out how people's lives really are for them and to respond appropriately (e.g., what they can afford, family food preferences, is their eyesight adequate to read labels, what equipment do they have in their kitchen), as well as encouraging people to be inquisitive about today's food products, is all part of the health promoter's role, that of empowering the individual to make sound dietary choices and decisions. Being up to date and fully cognisant of dietary concerns raised in the media makes the health promoter's role apropos the 'self-care' dimension immensely challenging.

Focus 2: mutual aid

It is frequently felt by individuals that they have little control over many of the factors that determine their health, including the availability, accessibility and affordability of healthy foods (Kemm and Close 1995). However, the efforts people make to deal with their health concerns by working together, could involve people supporting each other emotionally, sharing ideas, information and experiences (Epp 1986). This mutual help may emerge within a family, a neighbourhood, from a voluntary organisation or within a self-help group.

The Peckham experiment, though professionally-led, but in a low-key fashion, which brought a neighbourhood in London together and offered a sense of community, considered wholesome nutrition to be a central concern (Scott-Samuel 1990). More recently, the notion of community gardens and co-ops has been developed so that nutritious foods can be grown or purchased at a lower cost. Health visitors and other members of primary healthcare teams become increasingly active in the promotion of dietary health, directly (e.g., Spens 1996) or indirectly along the lines highlighted in the Ottawa Charter (WHO 1986), for example by enabling others to develop relevant personal skills and by facilitating community action.

How a group of women in Bolton tackled the problem of food costs is described by Jackson (1992). Funded by the 'Look After Your Heart' scheme, they set up a co-op with the intent to buy food in bulk and ultimately this led to the setting up of three other co-ops in other parts of Bolton. All of the targets chosen related to major health problems, namely common causes of

91

death or major illnesses, such as cardiovascular disease. Chosen targets had to be both achievable and capable of being monitored.

Included were risk factors relating to diet, such as obesity and saturated fatty acid intake (e.g., Kemm and Close 1995). Albeit somewhat restricted in nature, dietary health promotion had been identified as a government, and thus a national, concern. Nevertheless, the 'health of the nation' programme has been criticised for its leaning towards 'victim blaming', in other words that people are considered primarily culpable for their health problems. Possibly a broader approach would be more pertinent, one which clearly acknowledged, and addressed, the important part that the government and other public and private organisations have on making healthy dietary choices the easier choices for individuals and their families.

Epp's framework for health promotion

A pivotal question is: How does one set about promoting sound nutrition in the late 1990s? It is helpful in this regard to look back at the ideas of Epp (1986), a Canadian Minister for Health and Social Welfare, who envisaged health promotion as an integration of ideas from several arenas: public health, health education and public policy. His work is closely linked to ideas in the Ottawa Charter for Health Promotion (WHO 1986) and the WHO's goal of 'achieving health for all', as discussed in preceding chapters.

Epp suggests three mechanisms in his framework for health promotion which can be used to address health challenges:

1 self-care;
2 mutual aid;
3 creating healthy environments.

He also delineated the health challenges facing Canadians, and advocated increased social contact for many of the women as well as the exchange of recipes and cooking skills, which was particularly helpful for the younger women with families. At first, this project was hindered by too many professionals offering advice. However, in one town, the results of a survey, in which local, unemployed, single mothers were involved from the beginning to the final analysis of findings, led to the setting up of a community cafe. The importance of diet had been highlighted as a major influence on the health of the local people. In time, these women became recognised as 'advocates for local peoples' views, and as 'experts on health and diet' (Eaton 1994).

Labonte (1989), a health promotion officer in Toronto, discusses the importance of health professionals surrendering their 'service provider' need to control when involved in health promotion activities. It is urged that, instead, they should adopt a role of co-operation, aiming to empower others, rather than to colonise them with their own health agenda. Labonte helped to empower a group of low-income, single mothers in a Toronto housing project, and he described how he became a health resource to these women as they identified their problems. Basically these involved a lack of control over, rather than a lack of knowledge about, food. They could, therefore, confront their problem by organising 'pick-your-own' farm trips, community gardens and community dinners.

By a way of contrast, consider a study initiated by the Health Education Authority (1989) aimed to review the appropriateness of their literature on dietary advice for people on low incomes. While this exploratory, fact-finding study produced much more useful and descriptive information, it did little to engender a sense of empowerment. Rather it emphasised the respondents' plight without encouraging them to question their situation and identify underlying issues (Caraher 1994).

Focus 3: healthy environments

The third mechanism suggested by Epp, that of creating healthy environments, may be considered to be the most all-encompassing as it relates to the alteration or adaptation of our social, economic and physical surroundings in a way that helps to preserve and enhance our health. Even though people as individuals, and in some small groups, might wish to change their dietary behaviour and strive in unison with others to promote healthy eating possibilities, they have little power to influence the food giants and major international organisations involved in the food-chain. Government, which is ultimately responsible to its voters, holds immense power, both directly (e.g., legislation) and indirectly (e.g., regulation of trade and control of labelling and advertising) over people's dietary behaviour and choices. Ultimate decisions relating to the safety and quality of food as well as international trading standards are increasingly in the control of organisations such as the European Union and the World Trade Organisation (Lobstein 1994). Indeed the Government is expected to be concerned for the welfare of the people it serves, but this is not to say that it will necessarily act on adverse findings, for example regarding phytoestrogen levels in infant soya milks (Lobstein 1995).

Public outrage or dread may carry some influence, but current biotechnology is heavily guided by economic and political imperatives (Geary 1996). Increasingly, the patenting of agricultural biotechnology is being taken over by the large agro-chemical giants of the industrialised world, with lessening likelihood of such technology being used to provide cheap products for poorer nations (Pearce 1996). It has been said that we live in times when maintaining a good food supply for western nations, a task about which little mention is made in the general literature, would seem to be at the expense of poorer nations, many of whom continue to face malnutrition. Indeed, one might gain the impression that government ministers are unreliable in the promotion of a healthy dietary environment for the British public. However, Burke (1994), drawing on his experience of chairing the Advisory Committee on Novel Foods and Processes, describes ethical concerns relating to biotechnology as being addressed with a sense of caring involvement. Despite this, the Royal College of Nursing (1991), in its response to the Government's *The Health of the Nation* document, recommends that government-sponsored organisations should make more effort to provide healthy food (e.g., in schools, hospitals and prisons), so that the nation might see that the Government responds to its own message about the connection between diet and health.

How can the fostering of dietary health promotion be mediated? Should, for instance, food giants be allowed to sponsor material that is clearly self-promotional on nutrition and food-related issues for the use in schools without some form of government accreditation? This is done in Finland, for example (Potrykus 1991). How can conflicting messages be avoided, such as the development of butter, sugar and milk mountains and lakes as a consequence of government financial support to farmers, despite government recognition that the consumption of these very foods can lead to obesity and an increased likelihood of cardiovascular disease and diabetes (see Robbins 1991)? Why is poverty, which hinders people from readily affording healthy foods (e.g., foods low in sugar, salt and saturated fats, but high in fibre content) in adequate amounts, not being addressed adequately (Robin 1991)? Recently the BSE crisis has added to the lowering of consumer confidence in the Government as the European Union demands further culls in British herds. More and more it seems to be *Which?* magazine, and not the Government, that offers a help-line for those concerned about the crisis and fearful for their own health.

An excellent example of a health promotion initiative is 'Heartbeat Wales', a project set up with the intent to reduce the level of cardiovascular disease in Wales. It aimed to build on existing networks and activities as well as developing new ones (Catford and Parish 1989). Stimulating the adoption of habits of good nutrition was but one aspect of this project. Included among its targets were improved food labelling and an increase in availability of 'health foods' in shops, workplace canteens and restaurants.

Nine health authorities in Wales were involved as were mass communication networks. A 'Choice-Change-Champion' process for promoting health was followed, and involved the promotion of 'will-power', 'skill-power' and 'spill-power'. Despite the fact that improvements in lifestyle, including dietary behaviour did occur, it is recognised that these will have to be sustained if changes in the dietary behaviour of the Welsh people is to be maintained (Smith and Roberts 1994).

The task of health promotion is huge and, while primary health teams countrywide are involved in working towards 'health of the nation' targets, and initiatives such as 'Heartbeat Wales' have achieved dietary improvements, non-government organisations such as the Food Commission constantly challenge the *status quo*. Surely, what is needed is an independent food agency which would be responsible for food safety, but without being compromised by the food industry. As things stand now, the Ministry of Agriculture, Fisheries and Food (MAFF) represents the consumer but also the meat industry and farmers countrywide. The promotion of healthy environments is particularly complex, but we need not render it impossible. Inequalities within Britain as regards dietary health are not discussed vigorously enough and often ignore root causes such as poverty. Surely, it is at this level, that dietary health promotion should especially be focusing.

9

THE ETHICS OF HEALTH PROMOTION

The role of ethics in the discourse

Ethics is that branch of philosophy, and it is necessary to remember it is a branch of philosophy, that deals with what might be called 'right conduct' of people toward one another in society. Looked at in that light it can be seen that ethical analysis is possible of any human enterprise. To carry out such an analysis really means that we have to have unequivocal, almost empirical, definitions of common 'moral' words that we use freely every day, words such as 'good', 'just', etc.

Philosophers get around these logistical difficulties by two general strategies. They use as *few* such 'moral value' words as possible, ruling out all synonyms, for instance. Thus 'right conduct' is a pattern of behaviour between people consciously aimed at maximising the 'good'. Obviously some people will think of 'good', say, in theological terms while others will argue that this is not necessary and that 'good' can be accounted for entirely in secular terms. But the point to appreciate is that the origin, significance and beliefs about what is 'good, makes no difference at all to its role in ethics.

There are at least two widespread misunderstandings about 'ethics' among health workers. Firstly, that ethics is a 'lawyers' problem and, in any case, is the preserve of elite professional groups. Secondly, that ethical issue only need to be considered in life-threatening or otherwise dramatic situations. This is very far from the truth, but to appreciate this one must first understand the role of ethical debate.

Structuring ethics

In determining 'right conduct' the basic question must be 'What are the rights of one party against the rights of another in some given situation?' Ethics is the discipline of 'thinking and reasoning about mortality', according to Rowson (1990), while Campbell (1993) states: 'Since the time of Socrates – who declared that "the unexamined life is not worth living" and was condemned to death for the sentiment! – ethics has always been correctly

96

regarded as a critical discipline'. The adoption of a critical stand, needless to say, does not entail merely passively standing outside of the action and muttering aphorisms. Rather it is to question, not knowing what the answer may be.

Over the centuries two classical schools of thought have evolved about how to examine ethical issues; these are 'consequentialism' and 'deontology'. Consequentialists examine a series of possible actions and assess the relative merits of each. On balance, they then try to choose which action will bring about the greatest good for the greatest number. Obviously, situations will sometimes arise in which this desired balance is difficult to reach and the decision has to become the object of open debate.

Deontology, on the other hand, is an approach to ethics that concerns itself only with 'right action', *per se*, without reference to the arithmetic of people's views. The deontologist has a duty to be on the side of 'good', to do what is 'right' or to see that the 'right' thing is done. Ellis (1993) comments that 'the problem with following a list of do's and don'ts is that it reduces the role of the practitioner to that of a puppet and it does not allow for responses to the complexities of individual or even common situations'. If, just to take an example, it is a duty to respect autonomy, how does this duty apply to the very young or even people in comas?

An alternative approach, suggests Ellis (1993), to the exploration of ethical dilemmas is to combine both consequentialism and deontology, that is, to consider the rights and wrongs of actions and simultaneously have regard for their consequences. That, in fact, is the criterion used by most ethics committees in the NHS. Of course, in any situation ethical decisions can be influenced by factors other than moral duties and responsibilities. Professionals and lay people will always be subject to the influences of their own cultural and religious beliefs as well as the social and political pressures of the day. As we shall see later in this chapter, that can lead to problems.

Instead, ethics concerns itself with recognising 'good' when it occurs, and with specifying criteria for bringing it about. With this end in view, philosophers have long recognised and agreed that 'ethics' shall be defined as being mediated in four ways. These are:

1   beneficence;
2   autonomy;
3   paternalism;
4   non-maleficence.

These will be discussed and clarified in the context of health promotion in this chapter.

Prior to doing that, however, it is necessary to keep in mind that, although ethics can be analysed with respect to any human enterprise, the manner in which the ethics concerned is evident in each case will be different. For instance, a big difference in the relevant ethics prevails between health education and health promotion. If one is concerned with making sure that people (a target group) actually acquire certain information, we concern ourselves firstly with deciding precisely what that information is, then we elaborate teaching strategies to transmit it to the target group and then we have to work out some method of measuring to what extent we have been successful in the transmission process.

That is, our aim is *successful transmission*. What the individuals in the target groups *do* with the information is their concern and not the health educator's, although the latter will probably have very strong feelings about the matter. The ethical issues are largely contractual. Is the health educator providing information which is true? Are members of the target groups able to assess this independently? Are the instruments of assessment (examinations, practicals, etc.) imposed on the target group by the health educator accurate in measuring how much of what the health educator has done has been effective?

Until the early 1970s, ethics was hardly mentioned in this kind of context. The authority of medicine was so powerful that only rarely would someone have the temerity to look at the product, say, 'health' or 'health education', etc., to ascertain its value. As Julian Hart points out in his book *Feasible Socialism* (1994), the prevailing attitude was that the patient felt 'grateful' that someone as important and as highly trained as a medical doctor was bothering to help him in his affliction.

It is only in the context of lay-people's growing awareness of their rights, not only as 'consumers', but in all sorts of ways, that medical people began to seriously and systematically start to keep track of the ethical dimension. Nowadays one can hardly move in the health field without having to justify one's proposed action to an ethics committee.

Now all of this puts health promotion in a most curious position. This will be explained in detail as this chapter unfolds but, basically, the problem is this: in health promotion we claim to be concerned primarily with the person's sense of autonomy (self-esteem, human dignity, etc.). Our superior knowledge about health issues might make it quite obvious to us that a group of people, who were seeking health promotion advice, were leading lifestyles that conflicted with elementary canons of health. How can we project the health promotion message in such a way as to enhance the recipients' empowerment without denying their right to reject our message?

Freedom not to comply

When penicillin was discovered it was seen as a new breakthrough. However, a study of paediatric patients who had been prescribed this drug for severe strep throats showed that, after the five days of treatment, 18 per cent of the patients were non-compliant and, after nine days, the number had risen to 45 per cent (Charney *et al.* 1967 as cited in Raven 1988).

Such findings may astonish the reader. However, they can rest assured that they are not at all unusual and that compliance with medically prescribed treatment is a rarity (Collier 1989 as cited in MacDonald 1994). The stern reality of the situation is that up to about a half of all patients are non-compliant with prescribed medical treatments (Conrad 1985). On top of this many important health-related recommendations are either ignored or are not properly carried out. It is somewhat surprising to find that this is the case even if the treatment is considered 'life-saving' (Kaplan De-Nour and Czaczkes 1972 as cited in Raven 1988).

What is even more amazing is the extent to which many healthcare professionals themselves, including the very GPs who innocently hand out hundreds of unfilled or subsequently improperly used prescriptions for medicine that end up collecting dust in bathroom cabinets, remain blissfully unaware of the extent to which patients do not follow prescribed instructions. Indeed, it is reported that one doctor, on discovering such scandalously poor responses to prescribed medication, went so far as to diagnose the presence of a new 'resistant disease' (Sackett and Haynes 1976 as cited in Raven 1988).

However, growing appreciation of the extent of 'non-compliance' has made it a subject of great interest. It has been estimated that about 4,000 English language articles have been published on the subject up to 1985 (Trostle 1989) and a further 4,000 have appeared on Medline up to 1990. Nevertheless, and in spite of the interest, investigations into the causes of 'non-compliance' have proved inconclusive.

Obviously, most healthcare professionals have become exasperated by 'non-compliance', for it leaves them worried about the effective outcome of healthcare initiatives. Unable to cope with the belief that they have failed the patient, many such primary carers consequently label non-compliant patients as 'difficult' or inaccurately blame them for failing to understand instructions (Ryan 1994). There have even been situations in which patients have been refused treatment when they did not comply with the wishes of the healthcare professional (Moore 1995). The growing emphasis on personal autonomy, however, in recent decades has witnessed changes in health politics. Individuals are increasingly encouraged to see themselves as active consumers, particularly with the introduction of the Patient's Charter (DOH 1991), rather than passive recipients of healthcare. Moreover, there have been increasing demands for information about medical treatments and 'today's patient' wants to actively participate in his own healthcare (Ryan 1994). This represents a transition in philosophy and means that, how a patient is cared for and treated, must be right not only by accepted standards of care but also in the light of broader ethical principles.

Ethics and the right of non-compliance

It is remarkable that we should ever have thought the issue straightforward. Instead, both the aim of healthcare and who controls the balance of power with it constitute morally complex issues. This implies that 'compliance' in healthcare must be regarded as a central problem in biomedical ethics. In this chapter, then, after the reader has been introduced to the principles of beneficence, autonomy, paternalism and non-maleficence the pivotal question is then raised: Whose health is it anyway?

Our previous discussions illustrate how and why the proponents of the biomedical tradition came to hold the point of view that they are the experts, that they know best and are prescribing treatments for the benefit of the patient. In the context of that model, all the patient has to do to ensure 'good health' is to comply. Such an outlook beautifully represents the principle of beneficence which refers to an action done for the benefit of others. For healthcare professionals beneficence is a moral obligation (Beauchamp and Childress 1994) and this is even noted in the writings of Hippocrates, 'As to disease, make a habit of two things, to help, or at least to do no harm' (Jones 1923 as cited in Beauchamp and Childress 1994).

The injunction 'to do no harm', of course, represents non-maleficence. Independent arbitration, especially from outside of the 'profession', has only recently been recognised as feasible and, pretty well throughout history, physicians have been able to rely on their own judgements when it came to what was best for patients and how best to meet their needs. But beneficence is not the only criterion. Healthcare professionals are also obliged to provide the benefit (beneficence) without producing harm (non-maleficence). As a consequence, many doctors have felt compelled to coerce the individual into complying with their directives, so that their physical health improves, i.e. so that the non-maleficence aspect is satisfied. Despite the figures quoted above to illustrate the degree of non-compliance, we must never lose sight of the fact that, even by the eighteenth century, the 'authority of medicine' (and with such a scant empirical basis for it) was so paramount that many patients persisted in obeying their doctor's orders even to their obvious detriment. The composer Mozart's final illness was characterised by episodes of acute colic. His doctor had prescribed an antimony/mercury mixture. Not unsurprisingly, whenever the medically compliant Wolfgang took his medicine, the pains worsened. But his faith in medicine was so strong that he took this as an indication that he should take more. If only he had not been so compliant, he doubtless would have completed his C Minor Mass!

We have advanced since Mozart's time and now there is a common belief that the idea of providing healthcare purely through traditional healthcare philosophy is inadequate for present health needs (Seedhouse 1988). Increasingly, doctors are watched by lay groups and it has become important to establish whose benefit and whose harm is likely to result from any proposed intervention. Even so, the idea that beneficence takes priority over other moral principles, primarily the principle of autonomy, although an ancient one, is still alive and kicking (Seedhouse 1988).

Autonomy can best be described as the individual being able to choose freely for himself and to be able to direct his own life (Seedhouse 1988). It is obvious from what we know of psychology, if not from common experience, that people do vary considerably in their manifest level of self-assurance, and even a high-level of self-assurance as a shield when the opposite is really the case. It is because of health promotion's concern with empowerment that autonomy comes into the picture. But it also must be remembered whole cultures vary between themselves in the degree to which they consider self-autonomy important. The ethical implications of such cultural differences are immense, as demonstrated in Chapter 14. In the context of the present discussion, however, let us assume a western milieu. Even then, autonomy is constricted by society's structures, such as medicine, law, social tradition, the autonomy of other people and individual circumstances.

One assumes that mature people, at the peak of their development, are in the best position to make genuinely autonomous choices and, because they have the capacity, the principle of autonomy tells us to respect those choices (Gillon 1994). When children are involved, it is considered justifiable to be paternalistic, on the ground that children are less likely to choose what is best for themselves. When it comes to adults, there is a presumption (often wrong) that they know what is in their best interests, so that respecting their autonomy and promoting their welfare through beneficence coincide. In this, we are not only guided by 'presumption' but by the whole edifice of 'right under the law'.

Despite this, however, it is interesting to note that within most definitions of health, autonomy is not specifically mentioned. What better example could be afforded than the WHO's definition of health, expressed as 'a state of complete physical, social and mental well-being, not merely an absence of disease, illness and infirmity' (WHO 1986).

It is, of course, not difficult to criticise the definition on a variety of grounds. For instance, some commentators find the definition too restrictive upon which to base actual healthcare practice, because human value is not addressed. Altogether, according to Seedhouse (1988), the epistemological problems within healthcare stem from confusion surrounding the meaning of 'health' and it's link to human value. Human value, if one likes, relates 'autonomy' and 'dignity'.

John Locke (as cited in Seedhouse 1988) examined human value and what it means to be a human being. He argued that the central feature of human value was an awareness of a 'reasoning process': self-consciousness, whereby an individual can consider that he/she is himself/herself. Not only must one consider oneself as an entity, but one must 'value' oneself (Harris 1985). Such analysis led to Harris' definition of a 'person' as, 'any being capable of valuing its own existence' (Harris 1985).

While it can be argued that this definition produces appreciation of the basic concept of a person, it does not establish the essence of being a valuable living thing. Accordingly, Harris tried to extend his definition to encompass this aspect, in that individuals have the capacity to value their lives because they know their lives hold future choices. That is certainly one way around it. Hence, in order to consider the ethics of healthcare, the individual must be able to make his/her own choices (Seedhouse 1988). But here we come around full circle, for the ability to make choices for oneself is based on and presupposes the principle of autonomy (Gillon 1994).

Evidently, then, autonomy is an integral part of health, and all healthcare professionals must needs focus their work on this aspect. But this immediately raises a problem. Healthcare professionals believe, through beneficence, that they have the moral right to give priority to the principle of non-maleficence over the principle of autonomy, in order to 'save the patient from themselves'. Such a view of the patient's role is bound to the paternalistic concept of the 'doctor–patient' relationship, even when it does not lead to illegality. That is, when most healthcare professionals mistakenly believe that they recognise autonomy, it is in fact paternalism that directs their interaction with the patient (Coy 1989 as cited in Moore 1995).

Paternalism is defined as the intentional overriding of one person's known preferences or actions by another, and the person who exerts their preferences does so, ostensibly, in order to benefit or avoid harming the person who is overridden (Beauchamp and Childress 1994).

Therefore, while it is true that any patient suffering a long-term illness, can be considered to be an expert on 'their disease as it affects them', the healthcare professional is considered to be the expert on 'the disease itself' (Anderson *et al.* 1991). Such an explicit idea of paternalism in this scenario is based on the principle of beneficence, whereby it seems entirely justifiable that doctors overrule patients' autonomy and expect them to comply with their treatment regimes on the grounds that otherwise the patients' health may suffer. Patient autonomy tends to be recognised to the extent that it would be reasonable to presume that doctors should allow patients at least to contribute to their own health care and, most especially, to the whole relationship between doctor and patient. It is unfortunate that healthcare professionals often reject patient 'interjections' as irrelevant because such interjection diverts the primary task of 'making a diagnosis' (Waitzkin 1989). Consequently, patients are unwilling to disclose their beliefs on illness in case they are viewed as ignorant or irrational (Fitzpatrick 1989). Finally, the patients' perceived status of the healthcare professional adds to the already imbalanced interaction, whereby patients often promote the paternalistic relationship by agreeing to comply with medical directives (Strong 1979).

As O'Neill (1984) noted, although paternalism has benevolent motives, it does not always achieve beneficent results. Consider the case, for instance, of what happens when the healthcare professionals are involved with patient-based drug trials. For the healthcare professionals, both funding and reputation are major issues in such a situation. In that context, then, the normally 'neutral' paternalistic attitude must become 'non-paternalistic' (Beauchamp and Childress 1994).

However, paternalism may be disempowering and often is. In such situations it prevents the individual from acting autonomously and perverts the principle of beneficence. The chief ethical issue, to which both paternalism and autonomy are related, is that of informed consent (Faulder 1985). But consider what this implies. Informed consent has been defined as:

> the patient's rights to know, before agreeing to a procedure, what the procedure entails: the hazards; the possible complications; and the expected results of the treatment. The patient must understand any alternatives to the procedure, including in most cases, the results that can be predicted from non- treatment.
>
> (Holder 1981)

Non-maleficence

This, the fourth of the attributes of ethics, most commonly refers to the criterion that, having set out to exercise 'right conduct' by promoting the patient's 'good', the healthcare worker must not then do harm to the patient in order to achieve some object *other* than the patient's good. This may seem obvious, but actually it is astonishingly easy to find oneself in a situation in which maleficence arises. To convey to a patient the idea that what one is doing to him/her is for his/her good, when actually it is primarily for some other objective, certainly requires the exercise of paternalism. It can also be maleficence. In other words, such positive collaboration with the patient does not always occur. A startling incidence of this type of 'paternalism' occurred in diabetes healthcare management during the 1980s, when there was a complete changeover from animal insulins to 'human' insulins. It appeared to happen suddenly and there was certainly little discussion or information produced. As well, the reasons were commercial rather than clinical. There ensued reports from some patients of a loss or change in the hyperglycaemic warning signs they experienced. Incredibly, in many cases their concerns were ignored by healthcare professionals and the public was falsely informed that changing back to 'animal' insulins was impossible (Tattersall 1992). It subsequently transpired that some research suggested that the patient complaints were valid (Egger *et al.* 1992). It is even additionally alleged that the death of some patients occurred as a result of failing to recognise and treat hyperglycaemic episodes. If nothing else, this seemed to demonstrate that patient experiences and interpretations of their illnesses, even if different from those of the 'experts', are often significant (Morgan 1991). But confusion bedevils this area of paternalism for, although healthcare professionals believed they were doing the right thing for the patient, the patient had no control to do anything other than 'comply' with medical directives.

Clearly, some of the problems with paternalism are related to the shift in the healthcare professional–patient relationship, from patient-controlled to healthcare professional-controlled. Several analyses of the dynamics of this relationship have highlighted the importance of factors such as medical power and control (Parsons 1951), and this is reflected in the most commonly used definition of 'compliance'. That is, compliance is defined as the extent to which a person's behaviour changes in accordance with the advice or recommendations of some authority figure (Haynes *et al.* 1979 as cited in Raven 1988).

Conflict between autonomy and beneficence

Twenty years ago, Ivan Illich (1976) expressed this shift of power in terms of the 'medicalisation of life' and he stated that '(the physician) tends to mystify and to expropriate the power of the individual to heal himself and to shape his or her environment' (Illich 1976). Further, he suggested that the shift in power, and thus of control, was used for the benefit of the healthcare professional and not the patient. He summarised by averring that 'medicine' was used principally as a tool to maintain 'social control'.

The problems that all of this raise are not easily resolved. Respecting autonomy is a moral requirement, which means not interfering with an individual's decisions (Gillon 1994), but some authors believe that the principle of beneficence must take priority over autonomy. In their view, it is the healthcare professional's obligations to act for the patient's medical benefit and not to promote autonomous decision-making. Moreover, and possibly a different legal issue entirely, some argue that the presence of illness itself diminishes that capacity for autonomy and allowing patients to be involved in the decision-making process and providing them with too much information, in some situations could be of real harm (Pellegrino 1979). Commonly cited in this context is the issue of telling patients about the rare side-effects of prescribed treatments (Chadwick and Tadd 1992). Such situations occur with the best of motives and under the guise of beneficence, in other words, helping the 'sick' individual. But, in fact, health is linked to human value and thus the principle of autonomy and hence the contradiction. Should it happen that beneficence 'competes' with autonomy, be it under the banner of paternalism for the sake of non-maleficence, or not, then there will be disruption in the healthcare professional–patient relationship. In the final analysis, after all, patient power is exercised through 'non-compliance' (Gillon 1994).

Notwithstanding the foregoing argument, and in defence of beneficence against autonomy, Pellegrino (1979) argued that the healthcare professional's

104

duties are derived from an individual's choices. However, Beauchamp and Childress (1994) argue that it is a 'dressed-up defence of the autonomy model', and if the beneficence of healthcare professionals is based upon patient's preferences, then the principle of autonomy should surely assume priority over the principle of beneficence.

Those authors that believe the principle of autonomy ought to take precedence over the principle of beneficence argue that the healthcare professional's obligations to the patient in aspects such as disclosure, informed consent, confidentiality and privacy can most logically, then, be predicated on the principle of autonomy and not of beneficence (Beauchamp and Childress 1994).

The fundamental argument is most cogently expressed in John Stuart Mill's discussion of autonomy and paternalism, 'On Liberty' (1859), in which he pointed out that each person is the best judge of their own happiness and that autonomous pursuit of goals is itself a major source of happiness. Therefore, it is unlikely that interference by others could maximise this happiness. His belief was that autonomy was the essential requisite that allowed individuals to shape their lives and that individuals should be allowed to develop without interference so long as they do not harm or interfere with the freedom of others.

In an actual situation, it is understandable that with such a level of competitive beneficence, the patient would want some control. In many cases, as already suggested, non-compliance can be explained as an act of patient autonomy. Cannot one go further and say that it can be described as a deliberate attempt to reject advice and treatment, and to preserve a sense of autonomy (Grant and Mayande 1994)? Another real situation exemplifies the problem. It relates to measuring the levels of the drug, Phenothiazine, which has been found to be a very effective treatment for psychiatric patients. Naturally enough, on a closed ward, where compliance could be closely monitored, 93 per cent of these patients were found to be compliant. However, on an open ward, the non-compliance rate rose to 32 per cent and, for those on hospital leave, to 37 per cent (Irvin et al. 1971 as cited in Raven 1988). There can be no real doubt that, in this situation, non-compliance can be argued to be an act of self-determination by the patient, who has been adequately informed and advised, and in which the costs and benefits of a medically-prescribed treatment regime are weighed up and an individually 'tailored' package is produced to fit in with their psycho-social context.

Assessing the seriousness of non-compliance

Kelleher (1988) noted this aspect of autonomy. The study concerned focused on an examination of non-compliance and coping strategies in diabetic patients, and discovered there was a high-level of non-compliance. He felt that this had occurred because of the juxtaposition of the strict demands of treatment and that, at least in the short term, diabetes is not usually a painful or life-threatening illness. Amazingly, despite medical knowledge of the rates of diabetic complications that do occur with poorly controlled diabetes and despite all of the intensive patient education that is provided, patients still exercise their rights by adapting the treatment regimes to suit their lives. This illustrates the 'empowerment' difference between health education and health promotion rather well. To patients themselves, 'compliance' is rarely an issue at all and obeying orders, power and control issues are irrelevant. Holm (1993) goes so far as to argue that 'non-compliance' cannot actually exist as morally the relationship between the healthcare professional and patient must ultimately allow the patient, who has been adequately informed and advised, to make autonomous decisions. If that be the case, he/she cannot be described as non-compliant. One could describe such a person as foolish, obstructive and non-collaborative if he/she blatantly disregards decisions to which he/she is party, but as these remain a patient's own decisions and cannot be a doctor's orders, 'compliance' cannot be an issue.

We must be prepared to recognise, however, that there is a fundamental difference between the patient who has deliberately chosen not to take a healthcare professional's advice and a patient who has failed to grasp the implications of not acting on such advice (Grant and Manyande 1994).

It is essential to differentiate in ethical terms between deliberate rejection and what is described as benign neglect. To do so requires detailed consideration of why advice should have been rejected and it is necessary to understand the patient.

Benign neglect

For example, it is often the case that benign neglect reflects a personal belief system. One has only to consider the famous longitudinal study of all UK-born children in the first week of March 1946 (Douglas 1960). Certainly there was a strong association between poor educational achievement and parental attitudes, which were reflected in maternal behaviour such as poor uptake of antenatal services, poor maternal care and showing little interest in the child's progress at school. Moreover, Douglas believed these behaviours were at least in part a consequence of social and educational background.

Consider Davies' study (1991), which investigated the mortality rates of women with diabetes mellitus. It was noted that deaths were five times higher for women in social class V than for those in social class I and the study inferred that 'benign neglect' was a consequence of low social class. By way of contrast, according to Blaxter (1990), apparent associations between social class and health are primarily one of low income and health. As well, Wilkinson (1980 as cited in Blackburn 1991) noted how changes in income correlate with changes in health. For that set of reasons, then, disadvantaged families will suffer from poorer health, be it through benign negligence or other factors. Of course, it is well recognised that, for many illnesses, there is a 'skewed' distribution across social class in terms of standard mortality rates, yet most authors agree that inequalities within health and education resources are more to blame than anything else. Davies (1991) has been emphatic in promoting the view that education was the vital key necessary to reverse this trend. While in many cases this is undoubtedly true, such statements masquerading as respecting autonomy in fact still 'smack' of paternalism. In this we come face to face with what is probably one of the most difficult areas for healthcare professionals. They may even fail to realise that social and material inequalities exist and therefore that health inequalities also exist. Evidently, in such situations, it is changes in the social structure that will then benefit the individual.

What must be concluded, this author would posit, is that, when exploring ways to maintain the health of the individual in an ethically correct manner, it becomes necessary to examine the structure of society and how health exists within it. Ginzberg wrote, 'No improvement in the health care system will be efficacious unless the citizen assumes responsibility for his own well-being' (Ginzberg 1977).

This, of course, presupposes a proactive engagement in health promotion. The author would argue that no improvement in health will be efficacious unless the individual is allowed to assume responsibility for his own health in an 'equal' society and ultimately it is his/her autonomy that should be respected at all costs. In reality, individuals already do make their own decisions, whether these comply or fail to comply with medical directives. Nevertheless, it would appear evident that some aspects of autonomy and beneficence can be counterproductive, especially if autonomy is represented in the negative aspect of responsibility and takes the form of 'blame'.

This whole issue of responsibility has been fruitfully discussed by Brickman (1982 as cited in Yeo 1993). He distinguished two forms of responsibility: blame, defined as the responsibility for the problem; and control, defined as the responsibility for the solution. Four different combinations of these two forms can be represented as four different models, namely:

1   blame with control;
2   blame with no control;
3   no blame with no control;
4   no blame with control.

It is the final point which is the empowering one and which provides a sense of autonomy that 'collaborates' with beneficence. Although paternalism and non-maleficence are relevant in healthcare and health promotion ethics, they do remain secondary to the patient's wants. Regarded in that light, it is not too great an exaggeration to say that, if healthcare professionals continue to dominate the healthcare professional–patient relationship, then surely it is the doctors and nurses who can be accused of 'non-compliance'.

As Moore (1995) himself states, 'Collaboration, indicates a two-way street for information and mutual support; compliance is a dead-end street'. This relationship should be balanced, for it to be ethical, because if we are moving away from this towards a healthcare system that respects the autonomy of patients and their right to make their own decisions regarding their health-care, then the concept of compliance must be replaced by the concept of collaboration.

10

HEALTH PROMOTION AND
THE MASS MEDIA

Power of media

It would be difficult to overrate the significance of the media in modern industrialised nations. Media images pervade many aspects of western society, and it is imbued with the power to reinforce opinions and may indirectly influence attitudes and beliefs. It is its affect on, and the creation of, health beliefs that we shall consider in this chapter, both for individuals and within the wider arena of society itself. The mass media will first be considered as a commodity then be examined in terms of how they become used as an avenue for the dissemination of health information, with particular reference to health promotion. With respect to the latter, its role in advocating, motivating and informing are pivotal (Egger and Timsett 1993). It has been cogently argued that in today's society the media is integral to culture and television the drug of the nation. It is the educational potential that renders the media such a likely vehicle for health issues. With communication as a central aspect of health promotion, the media presents the opportunity of mass communication.

The media are the means by which information or entertainment are diffused. Marshall McLuhan's famous aphorism 'the medium is the message' can be quoted to stress that any medium, because it is an instrument, modifies our hold over the world and consequently our interpretation of experience (Sorlin 1994). What remains unquestionable is the influence of the media. Gerber (1992; cited in Wallack *et al.* 1993) observed that 'Today for the first time in history, most stories are not told by parents, schools, churches, communities, or even native countries or cultures, but by a handful of business conglomerates that have something to sell'. This is an important aspect to consider and often determines how 'newsworthy' an issue is, and may in turn determine the coverage an item may get. The driving force of finance may, of course, choose to ignore the need and public desire for health insight. However, it is vital to recognise that the 'mass media's ability to set the public agenda and amplify and lend legitimacy to the voices and views of our nation's political debates, renders them essential participants in social change of any kind' (Wallack *et al.* 1993).

Naturally enough, the mass media has been an object of educational research. An early model of it was the 'hypodermic model' (Rogers and Shoemaker 1971, cited in Tones 1990). In this model it was thought that the mass media exerted a direct affect on the mass population at which they were targeted. The media message was, as it were, injected into a passive community: if the message had limited effects, then there are two solutions, either an increase in audience exposure through the increasing size of the hypodermic or a different message (or serum) is needed (Tones 1990). There has been much evidence to discount this model. This is most notable in areas of complex behaviour change, such as modification of sexual behaviour and drug use. An alternative is Katz and Lazarsfield's (1995) 'two step theory' or the general body of Communication of Innovations Theory (Rogers and Shoemaker 1971; cited in Tones 1990). The Elmira and Decateur studies (Klapper 1961), in contrast, aimed to determine under what conditions the media best exert their effects. Furthermore, there is a modern view derived from the analysis of the literature which encompasses education, persuasion and influence (Aitken 1985). In theory this suggests that the media can be used for health promotion only under certain circumstances (Egger and Timsett 1993).

The appropriateness of mass media as a vehicle for health promotion or as generators of health insight is subject to debate. Since the 1970s it has gained increasing popularity as a strategy for delivering preventive health messages (Lau et al. 1980; cited in Redman et al. 1990). It has, as well, been noted by Redman et al. (1990) that mass media programmes appear to have a number of advantages over traditional public health strategies. These include the ability to reach a large proportion of the population.

Although it is important to bear in mind that the audience is a select one, studies have shown that those at higher risk are less exposed than low risk groups to health promotion messages and are more likely to forget the message (Bakdash 1983; Bakdash et al. 1984; Ben-Sira 1982; Dembo et al. 1977; Griffiths and Knutson 1960; cited in Froberg et al. 1986). This, therefore, renders it imperative to recognise that certain groups of the population are vulnerable in the sense that they are less accessible one way or another, especially given the inaccessibility of traditional medical delivery. Attempting to analyse this, Pierce and Daveluy (1986) examined the demographic statistics of viewers of media campaigns and found that they are reasonably representative of the general population. Moreover, they include groups, such as young males, who are difficult to access through such traditional avenues as general practitioners.

Perhaps more to the point, mass media interventions are a relatively inexpensive method of exposing the population to health information. The mass media can make use of 'visually potent images' to invent a hard-hitting and powerful message which is more often than not available to other avenues. 'Finally mass media are said to have the potential to modify the knowledge or attitude of a large proportion of the community simultaneously, thereby providing social support for behaviour change not available within individually targeted interventions' (Redman *et al.* 1990). Such social support has been found to constitute a vital ingredient for producing and maintaining behaviour change.

When the media get it wrong

As this chapter hopes to make plain, the mass media have immense potential as part of the intersectoral apparatus in promoting health and in enhancing both community and individual empowerment. This must not blind us, however, to the fact that mistakes do from time to time occur in the media's presentation of health messages. It is instructive to analyse this phenomenon, and one actual example of such a fiasco will be examined here, not with the object of trivialising the media, but of indicating the mechanisms that might be invoked to limit the damage when mistakes do occur.

It goes without saying that the author had ample choices of incidents on which to draw in this respect, but finally decided on the media coverage of research on the link between regular ingestion of aspirin and protection from heart failure. It deeply penetrated public consciousness in the US (where it had its origins), Britain and the entire industrialised world in less than a week, and still resonates widely in the public's health beliefs. Moreover, in this case, the media did not only play a subsidiary role, they actually were exclusively responsible in promoting a message opposite to that originally suggested by the research in question. Retro-analysis seems to suggest that one procedural misunderstanding in the use of a normally reliable fail-safe mechanism lay at the root of the whole uproar.

Many scholars have written about the case in question, but this account is derived from an analysis by Molitor (1993). The misreported research in question was carried out by Relman and published in the prestigious *New England Journal of Medicine* (*NEJM*) (1988). Like all their major medical journals, the *NEJM* had a policy giving the media advance copies of potentially newsworthy health items three days prior to formal pre-publication release. The purpose of this was to allow interested people in the medical community the opportunity to raise any objections that they might have. The fail-safe mechanism which is then intended to operate is as follows. The media, for their part, agree not to disclose details of the study concerned for another forty-eight hours so that journalists have time to interpret the details without worrying that some rival journalist will 'scoop' them.

However, as we were constantly reminded during those dreadful days of nuclear brinkmanship, even the best fail-safe mechanism can go wrong. In this instance, a journalists' agency broke the story after only four hours, because the time and dateline was misread due to a fuzzy printout! The consequences were immediate and enormous.

As a result of the story's release, the public knew all about it before the medical establishment did, for the latter are not accustomed to looking to the mass media for professional up-dates. Chemist shops (or 'drug-stores', as they are called in the US) were inundated with people buying bottles of Junior Aspirin and stocks were quickly depleted. In Britain, the same news item was reported on BBC Radio and then it hit both the tabloids and the broadsheets only a few hours later. Here, too, Junior Aspirin suddenly became an item in great demand.

Some medical subscribers received their copy of the journal up to a week later, therefore making it difficult for them to comment at a local level to their patients. This caused great frustration and many complaints to the journal. With regard to the way the press handled the story, it had both a commercial and public health importance. The top five US national newspapers ran the story with four of them putting it on the front page. Aspirin manufactures began advertising campaigns with ultimately ten of them promoting aspirin as a treatment for heart disease. Molitor compared the information relating to the aspirin research which appeared in the top five newspapers in the US with the formal aspirin study research report and the editorial by Relman. What is not clear is whether the press had access to the study research report or just the editorial, but it appears to be the latter. Without more information about the differences between the two publications, it could be questioned as to whether the journalists, if they did not have access to the report, may have related the study findings differently. Molitor himself wrote to the medical professionals cited in the newspapers to determine whether they had been misquoted to provide additional data for evaluating the accuracy of the journalist's story. The last aspect could well be affected by the social and emotional issues surrounding the story and doctors' personal accounts may vary depending on how the story affected them and the response they received from their quoted statement.

Most of the actual errors that Molitor found in the media résumés of the research were errors of omission and they related principally to the experimental subjects, who were all doctors. Largely unreported was what sort of men were excluded from the study and why. In fact, the reasons for not being included in the study were of key importance and none of the five major newspapers studied told their readers that doctors who agreed to take part in the study were kept from doing so if they had a history of heart attacks, strokes or cancers etc. Sixty-three per cent of the initial group of doctors who agreed to take part were eventually excluded because of such reasons. Molitor quotes examples of how this information was omitted or avoided by journalists who used words such as 'low risk group' or 'healthy'. Lay readers may interpret these two descriptions very differently or identify themselves with these 'groups' when they may be at a higher risk of disease, etc. than they thought. Indeed, the *New York Times* even defined healthy as not already taking aspirin.

What the study showed versus how it was described

The original report found that more strokes occurred in the treatment group taking aspirin and does acknowledge that it may also have other negative health effects. There was a 15 per cent increase in the number of fatal and non-fatal strokes in this group although it was not found to be significant, but when the data was subdivided by type of stroke and severity, there was significance. Naturally that was enough to concern the researchers and, weighing up the benefits of reduced heart attacks against the risk of gastro-intestinal bleeding and strokes, it was felt that taking aspirin to prevent heart attacks could not be routinely recommended.

However, other omissions related specifically to this point. Two newspapers omitted the finding that more strokes occurred in the treatment groups and only two warned the readers of the risks associated with aspirin use. One paper out of the five included both pieces of information. Serious omissions relating to medical quotes were also identified which changed the whole emphasis of the quote. For example, the editor of the *NEJM* was quoted as saying 'a milestone in the continuing struggle against heart attacks' when what he actually wrote was 'if the study's highly promising preliminary results withstand the test of subsequent full reporting and further peer review, the study will be regarded as a milestone . . . '.

Not all of the misreporting can be ascribed to honest error, however. Molitor found that journalists from the five newspapers sensationalised certain aspects of the study. The putative benefits of taking aspirin were described as 'standing out with unexpected vividness'. Research findings were also described as 'dramatic' and 'much greater than expected', etc. The aspirin study findings were, in fact, released three years ahead of schedule for many reasons, but this helped to sensationalise it within its own right. News of that study had been circulating throughout the medical profession with the potential for misinterpretation etc., as at that time it was felt the results were going to be significant in reducing heart attacks. This helped to add fuel to the fire and actually caused widespread misinterpretation. Journalists reported, though, that the benefits of taking aspirin are so great there was no need to continue the study.

What the newspapers did not report was that the aspirin study population sample was not representative of the general male population. All men involved were doctors and smoked less than the average American male. Ultimately during the study there were eighty-eight cardiovascular deaths, but, if the sample had been comparable to the general male population, 733 would have been expected. Because of these variables which affected the aspirin study results, Relman stated that 'a final judgement on the use of aspirin in apparently healthy subjects cannot yet be made with any confidence'. The newspapers manipulated the term healthy and used it when generalising that aspirin could be used by all of their healthy readers. Terms such as 'healthy' and 'healthy hearts' were used in inferring that it was suitable for those people to take aspirin. The *New York Daily News* (1988) printed 'the new research is the first to show that aspirin is good for those whose hearts are outwardly healthy'. Headlines such as 'Aspirin halves your risk of heart attack' and generalisations like 'some women', 'most healthy middle aged men' and 'women with risk factors' helped to increase the thought that taking aspirin would help the majority of the population. *USA Today* was found to be the most misleading paper in relation to this.

The aspirin manufacturers went on to advertise their products in a very positive light in relation to the study results. One advertisement stated 'this may be the most important ad you'll ever read' and 'aspirin could save thousands each year' and linked the products to a 'major new study'. Within one month the pharmaceutical and trade legal bodies had ensured that all the manufacturers had agreed not to promote their products in this way.

Generally, in the US, the criteria for reporting health risk are based on the legal idea of what a 'reasonable person' might be expected to think or do. Klaidman (1990) states that the 'reasonable reader' should be able to assume a report to be complete, objective and accurate and that it must be 'understandable'. Of course, journalists may have a limited scientific knowledge and interpretation may be difficult of some medical/scientific reports and inaccuracies can result from incomplete understanding. Interestingly, Molitor does not acknowledge the fact that journalists want to write stories that will sell papers and this, however we may not wish to think of it, can affect the material produced.

Although it is clear that the newspapers were at fault for inaccurate reporting and therefore for promoting incorrect health messages to the general public, not all the blame should be placed on the shoulders of the journalists. Copies of the *NEJM* are sent out with no accompanying press release which in cases such as this may have helped. Press releases which rank information by importance could help to reduce the incidence of research being misinterpreted and of it being taken out of context. This is a very valuable point. As a general rule, the medical profession tend to avoid the press, saying nothing rather than to risk being misquoted, etc. Possibly, the more the medical profession get used to dealing with the press, the more the lines of communication should hopefully improve.

Efficiency of the media

However, the role of the media in initiating widespread and long-lasting behaviour change may be overrated. Some communications experts have concluded that, although mass media may increase knowledge, they are ineffective in changing attitudes and behaviour (Flay *et al.* 1980; Griffiths and Knutson 1960; Peterson *et al.* 1984; Plant *et al.* 1979; Wallack 1981; cited in Froberg *et al.* 1986). Klapper's classic review in the 1960s of the effects of mass media stated that reinforcement of opinion is the main influence of mass media. The most effective means has been shown to be a 'supplementation with personalised approaches' in order to change attitudes and behaviour (Koskela *et al.* 1976; Lazarsfield and Merton 1975; Maccoby *et al.* 1977; cited in Froberg *et al.* 1986). To maximise the uptake of the message, full audience attention is essential. This involves the principles of targeting audiences with particular emphasis on 'hard to reach' groups. Most health promotion campaigns are based on the needs identified through research by health experts or government health authorities (Sirgy *et al.* 1985; cited in Egger and Timsett 1993). Thus, in order to focus effectively on clients' needs, 'segmentation' of the audience is required in order to manufacture appropriate strategies to reach them. This can take various forms, including the identification of risk behaviours, i.e. smoking, psychographic or lifestyle approaches and attitude or belief surveys (Slater and Flora 1989; cited in Egger and Timsett 1993).

There has always been pressure to focus primarily on those aspects that are perceived as needing change, that is attitudes and behaviours. However, in accordance with the evidence discussed earlier, the effectiveness of the media in doing this is dubious. Rose (1993) with reference to Prochaska (1991) considered a staged approach to segmentation derived from his clinical work with cigarette and drug addiction. They state that mass media health promotion campaigns are most effective in the 'precontemplation' and 'contemplation' phases, that is, where the individual is not even considering changing an unhealthy behaviour or when they consider it, but not in the near future or as a priority item. With respect to the more 'hard to reach' segment of the audience at large, the issues of targeting and identification become paramount. This has to involve consideration of psychological factors, because reduced accessibility may be due to 'distrust of large government organisations, a sense of fatalism and poor cognitive processing skills' (Freimuth and Mettger 1990; cited in Egger and Timsett 1993). Thorough and comprehensive research on the particular issues of accessibility and responsiveness constitute the only way to break these barriers. However, it may be necessary in the re-evaluation to realise that the most effective use of the media in targeting these groups is in supplying them with the link information, such as helpline numbers.

Needless to say, it is important to make the distinction between the generation of health insight through the media, and more alarmist tactics taken by certain media in response to health scares which have financial gain as the primary object. The 'public' are now more aware of the notion of informed choices and increasingly expect accurate information through this channel. In ethical terms, the media therefore have a responsibility to the public to publicise these 'alarmist' issues but in terms which acknowledge propriety. This raises another issue and that is that there is also a distinction to be made between what is referred to as the *use* and the *role* of the mass media. People constantly argue that the media could be used more effectively. For instance, there is the argument that the mass media can contribute to the public debate about health issues versus the view that the media are a source of inaccurate information through the advertising and entertainment channels, thereby restricting the arena of public debate through the reflection of commercial interests. Vital to recognise are the social and political factors in health promotion which are often ignored by the media. Among these is usually an explicit statement about the link between health promotion and social change and public policy development (Wallack 1990).

The media as generating health consciousness

With respect to the effective use of the mass media as generators of health insight, two concepts are central: social marketing and media advocacy. Social marketing aims to influence people's behaviour whereas media advocacy is enlisted to influence the environment. Social marketing exists around the issues of integrated marketing principles with social-psychological theories aimed at developing programmes to promote positive health behaviours. As a concept it became well known after its use in community projects to prevent heart disease in both Finland (Puska and Dornbush 1985) and the USA (Farquhar and Fortman 1984). Social marketing on the other hand aims to limit or erase psychological, social and practical barriers to positive health behaviour. On this account it has been criticised as 'manipulative and ethically suspect' (Wallack 1990). It is also blamed for promoting simple answers to complex health problems and for disregarding conditions that give rise to and preserve disease. The situation is even more perilous in the context of developing countries because this method does not take into account important environmental issues. It has led to a focus on changing individual behaviours instead. Such clearly reflects a reductionist approach with a blurred focus on health as simply an entity affected by individual risk behaviours and presumably not influenced by the wider outreaches of socio-economics and the environment. However, this is in flat contradiction not only to health promotion but to marketing also. One of the fundamental aspects of marketing, and hence of social marketing, is an awareness of the total environment in which the organisation operates, and how this environment effects, or can itself be effected, to enhance the marketing activities of the company or health agency (Kotley 1988; Pride and Ferrell 1980; cited in Egger and Timsett 1993).

Media advocacy could be defined as the strategic use of the mass media for advancing social or public policy initiatives. In theory, it aims to include the public in policy generation and to increase their participation in the definition of the social and political environment as they relate to health issues. 'Advocacy is necessary to steer public attention away from disease as a personal problem to health as a social issue and the mass media are an invaluable tool in this

116

process' (Wallack *et al*. 1993). It is, however, beset by several limitations. These include the complexity of the skills involved. For instance, the media advocate needs to recognise what is 'newsworthy' and how it can be presented to stimulate both media and public interest. It demands a great deal of time for research and for networking those people who have access to the media. The media themselves seem to have a preference for personal and individual health problems, whereas media advocacy tends to focus on the environmental approach. It may therefore be difficult to retain the interest of the media and anything of a controversial nature may also induce hesitancy on the part of the media. Media advocacy helps to emphasise the importance of creating improved social conditions and is of value to those most in need, even though they are often those least able to change. Alternatively, social marketing is useful for developing the most creative ways of getting information to people and of overcoming barriers. Media advocacy makes use of unpaid publicity, whereas social marketing is usually associated with paid advertising, although neither are exclusive. Therefore, to maximise the use of the mass media in promoting health, the two strategies should be used concurrently (Wallack 1990). In some instances, of course, it has been found that individual-targeted campaigns must have first impact on beliefs and attitudes towards the recommended behaviour before socio-political advocacy objectives can be achieved (Egger and Timsett 1993).

It has been noted in the literature that there is lack of a systematic method for dissemination of research information and that this may have conferred a widespread superficial understanding of how the media can best contribute to health promotion. Unfortunately, such a limited understanding may also influence the practitioners' use of media-based intervention strategies (Flora and Wallack 1990). Following their study on the extent of media use for health promotion in California, Flora and Wallack acknowledged that the use of media was probably not as effective as it could have been and that future research should focus on translating research into practice. Contrary to the widespread belief of the pervasive nature of the media, reviews of research evidence usually conclude that the effects obtained are either relatively small (McGuire 1986a and 1986b), inconclusive (Freedman 1984) or contingent upon various conditions that limit the ability to make generalisations based on the results (Roberts and Maccoby 1985). Therefore, our primary concern must be not whether the media work, but under what conditions they can work most effectively.

Differential use of the media

To exemplify this point, consider the following. Three well-known studies were carried out in the 1970s which in essence were community health promotion trials on a large scale involving the mass media. They compared the impact of mass media only interventions with mass media plus community programmes with control communities that had no intervention at all. These were the Stanford three cities studies in the USA (Maccoby and Fenner 1977), the North Karelia project in Finland (Puska and Dornbush 1985) and the North Coast Healthy Lifestyle Program in Australia (Egger and Timsett 1993). Results showed the best combination to be the mass media plus community based programmes, although the mass media alone did have an impact. The success of the campaigns could be attributed to 'the extensive' use of formative research regarding audience and message variables and the supplementation of media with interpersonal communication within small groups that provide social support and modelling of appropriate behaviours (Solomon 1982, 1984; cited in Egger and Timsett 1993).

Thus, although the media may not be effective in altering behaviour directly, they may be able to supply motivation or awareness of a health problem which can later be expanded by other intervention strategies. This involves the concept of 'agenda setting', and has been shown to be effective in the mass media plus community studies discussed above.

Consider the 'Sydney Quit for Life' campaign (Dwyer et al. 1983; Pierce et al. 1986; cited in Redman et al. 1990). It was successful in using a wide range of media and repeated short professionally prepared media messages to encourage viewers to phone the quit line, which then provided practical information on stopping smoking. The results showed a significant effect on smoking with a decrease of 6.1–15.7 per cent on smoking prevalence in the intervention town (dependent on age and sex), while the change observed in the control town was only 2–5 per cent (Redman et al. 1990). Measurable changes in behaviour were also shown in the evaluation of a mass media led campaign to increase the compliance with Pap smear screening in an Australian study by Shelley et al. (1991).

It should be remarked, however, that although changes in behaviour have been shown to occur when the media have been used in an agenda-setting role combined with a community component, there is currently no evidence that the effectiveness of such combined programmes can be solely attributed to the media component. How do we know whether or not similar magnitude behaviour changes occur when the community component is used alone or linked with a cheaper method of agenda setting (Redman et al. 1990)? Redman et al. (1990) proposed that, in order not to discount the mass media strategy for altering health-risk behaviours, there needs to be a re-evaluation of researchers' skills, including a need for evaluation studies to formulate better methods of obtaining a representative sample and of validating their outcome measures. Statistical techniques would have to include the evolution of a theoretical and empirical core for designing media programmes; correlations of media plus community and community alone programmes and the attempt to design and evaluate media interventions which have greater community input and less involvement of marketing.

In large measure, it can be argued that promoting health through the mass media has ironically been developed from the notable success of the media in promoting unhealthy products, i.e. cigarettes, due in part to the huge funds now available for marketing. Those psychological processes used in advertising these products have been examined and utilised to develop, for example, anti-smoking campaigns. Of course, health is promoted by the media through various avenues, namely advertising, publicity and a more covert form is through what has been referred to as 'edutainment', that is, in messages integrated into fictional broadcasts such as soap operas. This avenue is perhaps of more benefit to those who could be classified as 'hard to reach' and who are unlikely to pick up a good broadsheet or to watch the *Nine O'Clock News*. There may also be more likelihood that they will retain the message when it relates to characters with whom they have some affinity. Related to this, the rationale for edutainment can be based on the social learning theory (Bandura 1977; cited in Maccoby 1980) whereby viewers will 'model' behaviours that they observe.

Edutainment uses media vehicles whose primary purpose is to attract a commercially viable audience and to achieve socially desirable changes in beliefs, attitudes or behaviours. It is a relatively new concept with the first international conference on the topic 'The enter-educate conference: entertainment for social change' being held in 1989. Of course, it can take various forms, including the deliberate co-operation between health and entertainment professionals to achieve a particular health goal and, in contrast, what has been referred to as the 'disease of the week' syndrome whereby controversial and newsworthy issues are dealt with in soap operas, etc., simply because of their topical nature. Again, such 'voluntary' treatment of health issues often tends to focus on individual aspects and to neglect important and relevant socio-environmental factors.

This phenomenon seems most prevalent in developing countries, where often television and radio are used to reach rural communities, using popular music to carry health and social messages. For this to work effectively, there must be a clear understanding of the potential mutual benefits. Health professionals have to strive to ensure that the messages are subtle. At the same time they need to realise that the commercial aspect is probably of primary importance to the media, who must in turn realise that the integrity of health promotion messages can enhance the appeal of a programme and ultimately reap greater financial rewards. Although this is obvious, it highlights the fact that in order to optimise the delivery of a message, the media and health professionals have to work in partnership.

The media and AIDS

Demands are constantly made on mass media by a huge array of public expectations, often fuelled by news items. These ultimately are balanced by the reigning hand of the Government, in Britain, and the commercial viability of 'the story'. When a health issue is highly topical and potentially controversial, the ethics of information giving, or not giving, come into focus as does the need to prevent the hysteria which often is attendant on such an issue. Clearly these are issues which can be vitally important and could save lives.

The HIV/AIDS campaign, which has been widely publicised, is pertinent to this discussion and highlights the effect of the media in the development of health policy. Virginia Berridge (1991) in her paper 'AIDS, the media and health policy', notes the significance of this disease and relates the press presentation of AIDS as central to the 'New Right resurgence' approach of the Government at that time. The reader will be well aware of the initial moral panic created by the tabloid press in their presentation of AIDS as a 'gay plague'. In fact, this somewhat overshadowed the relationship of the media in the establishment of 'consensual models of policy making'. The media portrayal of HIV/AIDS began in parallel with policy development and reflected the sexual sensationalism so popular with the press and, throughout its course, it moved on to include the issue of heterosexual spread of the disease and then through a phase of normalisation which resulted in the changing media attitude to AIDS as a scientific issue. All of this, however, should be seen in a framework of the interplay between different scientific constructions of the disease and their presentations to the public. Contemporary analysis of the media effect give currency to the idea that the press can only reinforce existing views and not change them.

Research (focused primarily on voting behaviour) has stressed that, as ties of class and community have loosened in the 1980s, the media have had a more autonomous relation to belief and attitudes (Harrop 1987; cited in Berridge 1991). It is important to note the distinction between the press and television presentation of the AIDS issue. The press, as noted earlier, reflected the New Right ideas of the government, whereas the television advertisements encapsulated the consensual model, with the main message being harm minimisation rather than morality. This highlighted the television as 'a more liberal consensual medium than the press' (Berridge 1991).

It is widely believed by lay people, of course, that celebrities have a role to play. Research, as well, has shown empirically that exposure to celebrities through the media can have an important influence on the public's health-related attitudes, beliefs and behaviour (Brown and Basil 1995). This was reflected in the LA Lakers basketball star 'Magic' Johnson's declaration that he was HIV positive and the extensive use of the declaration to promote HIV/AIDS prevention. Emotional involvement with Magic, through parasocial interaction, was important in mediating persuasive communication and results showed that a celebrity can effectively sanction health-related messages. There is, moreover, evidence to suggest that this celebrity involvement may have a more powerful impact on the public than does exposure to knowledge-based AIDS prevention messages themselves. The agenda setting influence of media coverage of the deaths of Arthur Ashe and Rock Hudson are likely to have contributed to an increase in public concern over HIV/AIDS (Rogers *et al*. 1984; cited in Brown and Basil 1995).

A careful epistemological analysis of the stages in the process of development in a health campaign, such as that for AIDS, in the progression from mass hysteria to the widespread publication of scientific fact, would be valuable. Increasing numbers of campaigns of this genre are currently running, with a notable focus on public participation through such actions as the wearing of coloured ribbons. For example, the breast cancer campaign has as its emblem the pink ribbon and October was marketed as 'Breast Cancer Awareness Month'. Ideally, the main focus of such campaigns should be accurate information giving, in tandem with a strong and powerful message highlighting risk and education on positive health behaviours.

The recent finding (*Sunday Observer*, 16 February 1997) that Britain has the highest incidence of teenage (15–19 years) pregnancy of any western European nation emphatically illustrates the potential for effective use of the media in promoting health awareness and rational behaviour. There is no shortage of issues on which to focus.

In conclusion, the mass media when used effectively, represents an ideal avenue for the delivery of health messages. Both the media and health promotion are strongly linked in their commitment to communication. The issue is complex, however, and it is vital to recognise the problems that exist in achieving a marketable message and the difficulties that beset this challenge. The media and health promotion are issues that answer to a number of differing 'authorities', most notable is the obligation to ethical practice and economic factors. In examining this issue the multifaceted nature of health must be recognised as paramount, the marketable nature of health be understood, and the media recognised as an invaluable tool in the promotion of positive health behaviours and reinforcement of opinions.

11

HEALTH PROMOTION IN THE CONTEXT OF EMPLOYMENT AND UNEMPLOYMENT

Work and health

Probably the most significant personal identifier of someone living in the industrialised world is what he/she does to earn a living. The link between the person, their social significance and sense of self-esteem and the particular paid work they do is doubtless less conspicuous in societies in the developing world. Reasons for this include the fact that, in less industrialised societies, paid employment is less differentiated and much of it labour-intensive agricultural work. But it is when the nexus between 'the person' and 'the job' is broken by unemployment that we notice how closely linked psychological health (self-esteem and self-actualisation) is to employment and how intimately this affects not just general health, but specific measurable clinical indices. Therefore, from its recent re-emergence in the 1970s and 1980s, health promotion and concern with it, has been perceived very much as an adjunct of the workplace in the developed world.

Historically, though, this is in marked contrast to the outlook which has prevailed with respect to health and work throughout almost the entire span of recorded history. Our greatest awareness has been with the extent to which we can accommodate work to survival. The dominant concern has been the relationship between work which must be done and its cost in terms of compromised health. One has only to read the Hammond books (1932), *The Village Labourer and The Town Labourer*, to gain an appreciation of how the story of the Industrial Revolution in Britain could be told almost entirely in terms of health and safety costs.

Advances in democracy in the industrialised nations and in attendant mechanisms of 'accountability' have recorded 'attitudes to work' as an important health variable. As health promotion is predicated on the exercise of autonomy, so also, from 1945 to 1980 in the UK, did we witness an increasing importance being attached to 'job satisfaction'. Unless jobs could attract people on the basis of job satisfaction, which automatically and psychologically carries a health cachet, they tended not to get done. In Britain this coincided with an influx of migrant labour, each wave of which tended to

122

take over the 'low job satisfaction' work which the previous wave had forsaken for something more personally fulfilling.

Indeed, one can trace a number of important changes in the workplace in industrial countries to the end of the Second World War, a convenient historical node for us because it provided the context for the emergence of modern health promotion. In this chapter, these more optimistic developmental links (say, from 1945 up until 1980 in the UK) will be analysed and a theoretical perspective developed. However, it is this author's contention that we can no longer regard the level of economic insecurity, which has become a paramount feature of the workplace since 1980, as a temporary 'blip' in an otherwise upwardly-bound situation. Unemployment, and insecure employment, are dominant features of the workplace scene in the UK today, and the role of health promotion in that context will constitute the major component of this chapter.

Populations have tended to become more affluent since 1945, and the culture of consumerism is gaining pace. Mass markets, now global, have become highly competitive and the industries supplying those markets have had to make profound changes in their organisations in order to compete. Previous methods of manufacture and even of industrial organisation proved inefficient, in respect of both production volume and in the maintenance of product quality. Moreover, even as industry has had to adjust to the commercial realities of a changing society, so also have those societies had to adjust to changes which, in turn, have impacted profoundly on the personal, social and working lives of their people. Hence today, in all sectors of industry, attitudes have either changed in response to these influences or are in the process of changing.

Psychosocial origins of attitudes to work

We realise now that attitudes generally are constructed from a number of complex and interactive factors and that these inform both our belief and our feelings about the world we inhabit. The cognitive component of attitude (the belief component) derives from our social interactions and from our experience of the environment in which we live. However, these experiences are not assimilated as purely objective bits of information, but also reflect the personal make-up of the individual, which is the mediating agent in the process of interpretation. Therefore, how we construct and feel about those beliefs is heavily dependent on our own particular psychological orientation, as well as on the objective realities giving rise to them.

There is considerable evidence that the nature of work plays a pivotal role in this. For example, Fukuyama (1992) has constructed a theoretical paradigm to argue that there is a certain inevitability about the process of social change which accompanies advanced industrialisation. A crucial feature of this process, he argues, is the need for universal education. It is obviously vital to invest in human resources to supply the know-how to sustain high-technology industry, and this is by no means a new idea. Drucker was also of the opinion, nearly thirty years ago, that the 'central capital of change . . . likely to mould and shape our tomorrow' in the arenas of 'economy, polity and society' is 'knowledge' (Drucker 1969). However, according to Fukuyama's thesis, the outcome of universal education is that it 'appears to liberate a certain demand for recognition that does not exist among poorer and less educated people' (Fukuyama 1992), and for Drucker (1969) there are the responsibilities of the new 'men of power, the men of knowledge'.

The dream, of course, is the rather unrealistic one of unrestricted growth. If the technological society is to realise the aspirations of 'limitless accumulation of wealth, and the satisfaction of an ever-expanding set of human desires' (Fukuyama 1992), then its social culture must become both liberal and democratic. Through a process of social evolution, he avers, this form of organisation has become the most adept at containing the 'liberated' population, and he predicts that it will become the natural political and economic destiny of the developing economies. Citing the western European and American democratic models as illustrations of the process, he states that consequences of liberalisation and democratisation are such that, as standards of living increase, and as populations became more cosmopolitan and better educated, society as a whole achieved a greater equality of condition, and 'people began to demand not simply more wealth but recognition for their status' (Fukuyama 1992). More succinctly, as life's experiences change, so do the expectations borne of those experiences.

In the US, Canton (1984) also describes a 'cultural transformation' of society, and he, similarly, attributes it to 'expanding human desires'. But his interest is in how the condition of 'expanding desire' is characterised. How it came or comes about is, to him, much less important and he suggests that there are three components; namely self-actualisation, androgyny and social actualisation. Self-actualisation, in fact, constitutes the highest attainment of Maslow's (1970) concept of the psychologically healthy person (as quoted by Nelson-Jones 1994). In health promotion terms we would describe such a person as 'empowered'. As a concept, it expressed the condition of the realisation of one's own personal meaning and creative potential and is dynamically expressed in the individual's need to take personal control over their life.

In organisational and sociological terms, and this embraces employment, Nelson-Jones also attributes a more democratic character structure and an increased identification with the human species to this level of personal fulfilment. One of the consequences of an increased level of personal responsibility and autonomy, Maslow also suggests, is the development of an attitude that he terms 'resistance to enculturation' (Maslow 1970; quoted by Nelson-Jones 1994).

Health promotion as context and consequence

Health is obviously pivotal to this because self-actualisation is rarely achieved, unless the basic hygiene needs of the individual are first satisfied, and it is assumed in Fukuyama's (1992) thesis that this condition is met by the economic affluence realised by the liberal industrialised economies.

The need for health promotion to transcend such marginalising agencies as racism and genderism is cogently reflected in this. Consider androgyny, for instance, it is in some ways analogous to 'feminism', which is perceived as the shift from sex-role stereotypes and the freeing from the social constraints which such a system imposes. A similar dynamic was seen by Johnson (1986) in the 'counterculture movements' of the 1960s and 1970s. This was particularly so among women and minorities, to which he also ascribes the accelerated emergence of the holistic health movements.

A necessary effect of this, of course, is the third component of Canton's (1984) self-actualised person, namely social actualisation. In health promotion, neighbourhood advocacy calls forth a growing recognition of the fundamental interdependence between individuals and their social institutions and of the need for individuals to satisfy their goals through participation and proaction, rather than by apathy and reaction. It was argued by Canton (1984) that the realisation of social accountability is inextricably tied to individual wellbeing. From a slightly different emphasis, this point was made earlier by Nelson-Jones (1994) and a significant amount of empirical evidence derived from organisational theory suggests that this is the case.

For instance, a study of lifestyles, which captured some of the attitude of the 'counterculture' suggested above, was conducted by Friedlander (1975), who observed that the pattern of youth reflects, *inter alia,* 'a strong preference and value for self-guidance, self-exploration, self-discovery based upon freedom to experience a variety of feelings and events'. His view suggests that youth 'seems to be turning away from the mechanistic organisational structure – not from organisational mechanistic – but from the mechanisation of man', and questions 'what implications might [these] preferences, beliefs, and values have upon future organisational structures...?' (Friedlander 1975).

Can the workplace accommodate health promotion?

As mentioned earlier, for reasons of survival, industrial organisation has had to change. But for organisational change programmes to succeed, it is necessary for the change agent to know something about the employees and to somehow accommodate to their needs, goals, values, interests and backgrounds for, as we have already argued, it is ultimately the cognitive and effective components of our attitudes which determine how we behave. For this reason, organisation theorists regard the formation of attitudes of singular interest as providing a means whereby they may gain an insight into the process of how their employees' beliefs are formed or influenced, how they feel about what they believe and how these beliefs and feelings translate into behaviour. Various theories have been proposed to explain the relationship between feelings, beliefs and behaviour.

One need only refer to such paradigms as Festinger's (1957) cognitive dissonance theory and Bem's (1967) theory of self-perception of how attitudes are influenced (both quoted by Rajecki 1990). Both have their proponents in industry. From another perspective, Dyer (1984) tends towards the former and considers that changing behaviour is personally motivated by, and results from, a fundamental shift in the personal belief structure: 'when . . . change occurs it is because some person has decided to alter his or her performance' (Dyer 1984). The intimately personal aspect is emphasised in that : 'change is intensely personal. For change to occur . . . each individual must think, feel, or do something different'. That is, both see change as an intensely individualistic phenomenon, what we would recognise as a component of the empowerment process.

Taking a somewhat different stance, Beer (1990), however, while accepting that behaviour is 'a function of individual knowledge, attitudes and behaviours', contends that changing behaviour is more significantly influenced by 'task alignment'. Task alignment tends towards Bem's 'self-perception' as a significantly influential factor in modifying behaviour. Indeed, it is suggested that 'individual behaviour is shaped by the organisational roles that people play' (Beer 1990). In this context, of course, attitude is inferred from the situation. It is the organisational context which imposes the new role.

Both self-perception and cognitive dissonance theory may be correct to some extent, depending on the particular relationships and organisations under scrutiny. However, we are amply justified, especially as health promoters, in asking what impact these insights into management theory have had on employment practice. In Britain, for instance, the growing positive link between developing insight into health promotion and increasing autonomy in the organisation of work practice, certainly reached a hiatus in about 1980. The 'market forces model' gained ascendancy and has by now become the cognitive arbiter in legitimising (or otherwise) commentary on health in the workplace. It would appear that the relevant question to ask today is: 'Does it lead to increased sales?' rather than 'Does it enhance the human dignity of the participants?' The most obvious reflection of this 'New Right' social thinking is the changed attitude toward unemployment.

Instead of regarding unemployment figures as a measure of a national economy's inefficiency, we are increasingly being asked to accept it as a necessary adjunct to economic viability.

Health promotion in the context of unemployment

Since 1981, the UK has experienced high-level unemployment. Some link this with the first oil price adjustments in 1974, for these brought recession that really signalled the end of the full employment of the post-war boom years. In the past twenty years unemployment rose to a peak of 3 million in 1986 and never dipped below the figure of 1.6 million (in 1990). In 1996 Convery quoted the most recent UK figures as showing unemployment dipping under the 2 million mark or 7 per cent of the working population. Moreover, these figures tell only part of the story. While economists regard unemployment as an economic cost in terms of loss of potential production, health promoters look to the social and individual costs of unemployment. Therefore, a focal point for this chapter is the link between unemployment and health. It is evident from a huge range of studies that continuing high unemployment has profound implications for the health of individuals and communities. Research conducted throughout the century points to an indisputable link between unemployment and poor health. Recent analysis is focusing on examining the psychosocial nature of this relationship. From an understanding of the causes of ill-health in the unemployed comes an appreciation of the measures that need to be taken to redress the balance and it is not hard to argue that the health challenges presented by unemployment can best be addressed from a health promotion approach. Out of all the differing approaches to health and healthcare, health promotion is best equipped with the theoretical perspectives that lead practitioners to ask questions about the social causes as well as effects of conditions because of its preoccupation with empowerment.

Attempts at empirical analysis of the problem are bedevilled by semantic problems. How do we define 'unemployment'? Widely used is the International Labour Organisation's definition that someone is unemployed if they are without paid work and are looking for a job. In Britain, the government figures include the number of people claiming state benefits and who are looking for work, the most recent innovation being the Jobseekers Allowance. Thus, differences in the way that unemployment is measured render it difficult to compare unemployment figures between countries and within countries over time.

Official unemployment figures in Britain are produced by the Department of Employment. But, it is claimed by the Unemployment Unit, an independent body, that the way that the figures are calculated has been changed thirty times between 1979 and 1990 and that twenty-nine of these changes had the effect of reducing the total number of unemployed. The Department of Employment itself admitted to only seven changes in the same period (Clark and Layard 1993). Clearly this has a political dimension which must be understood. For instance, recall the famous Conservative Party poster of the 1979 election campaign which showed a long queue of unemployed with the slogan 'Labour Isn't Working'.

And the unemployment figures themselves underestimate the social scale of the problem. For instance, women are underestimated in figures that count the unemployed male head of household as the only one unemployed in that family. Fagin and Little (1984) argue the obvious in that unemployment affects entire households and not merely individuals.

Empirical links between unemployment and health

A review of research conducted between the world wars reveals a contemporary interest in investigating whether poverty leads to ill-health among the unemployed. Constantine (1980) showed that several official reports all concluded that the effect of unemployment on health was minimal (Astor *et al.* 1972; Ministry of Health 1929; Owen 1932; all cited in Constantine 1980). Official analysis of the diet of the unemployed suggests that state and local government support payments were sufficient to provide a healthy diet. Even so, it was frequently found that women had poorer diets than men or children of their households, as they tended to sacrifice their own needs to those of others. At that time, of course, concern with the poor diet as the factor by which to measure health reflected a contemporary concern to show that national insurance payments, local poor relief, free meals for children all combined to adequately meet the dietary needs of the unemployed. Not surprisingly, Constantine's review of the contemporary evidence suggests that official responses were regarded as being complacent. Concern with the topic ended with the Second World War and remained forgotten as the post-war boom made unemployment seem an issue of the past. But a dramatic return to high unemployment in the 1980s was mirrored by renewed interest in the subject.

Research published since 1975 is unanimous in pointing to the clear conclusion that unemployment is statistically associated with poor health.

Empirical measures

The OPCS Longitudinal Survey produced results showing that unemployed men and their partners have a 20 per cent higher risk of mortality, even after other potential risk factors, such as occupational class, are accounted for (Moser *et al.* 1990).

Again, the British Regional Heart Study has also provided longitudinal study information. It was found previously that periods of unemployment during the study lead to significantly raised mortality after other factors have been excluded (Morris Cook and Shaper 1994).

Death can be regarded as an extreme form of ill-health, albeit a persuasive one! Mortality figures, however, do not give an indication of the actual health experiences of the unemployed. Beale and Nethercott (1987, 1988) have reported the changes in health of a group of workers made unemployed when a local factory closed. What they did was to ascertain that increased morbidity followed unemployment, as measured by increased use of GP and hospital services. Also, their research shows that the decline in health started when the news of the possible closure of the factory was first announced two years before the actual closure occurred.

Beale and Nethercott (1988) proposed that this finding indicated stress as the most significant factor. It has been argued that fear of redundancy is seen to be equal in stress value to the actual experience of unemployment. Prolonged unemployment must be a source of chronic stress. Unemployed people experience the feeling of loss of control over their lives. Baum *et al.* (1986) show that, while those who have recently lost a job exhibit stress patterns little different to those in employment, the long-term unemployed exhibit signs consistent with Seligman's theory of learned helplessness.

A number of other surveys have used self-reported measures of health. A good example is The Health and Lifestyles Survey, which used four indices to measure health: fitness based on physiological measurements; diseases based on medically defined conditions; experience of illness based on self-reports of symptoms suffered; and psycho-social wellbeing based on self-reported symptoms. On each of the four dimensions, the unemployed were found to have poorer health.

Naturally, the effect of unemployment on mental health has attracted many studies. Fagin and Little describe the loss of a job as being similar to a bereavement. Although the relationship between stress and physical illness is not fully understood, a broad definition of health would surely regard stress as unhealthy in its own right.

West and Sweeting (1996) studied the effects of unemployment on young people involved in a longitudinal study based in the Glasgow conurbation. They found that at the age of eighteen, the unemployed experienced significantly worse mental health than their peers while its impact on physical health was inconclusive. Interestingly, the study also reports a positive correlation between the expectations of future unemployment and poor mental health. In addition, it has been shown that depression and neuroses are also more common among the unemployed (Wilson and Walker 1993).

Analysis of the relationship between unemployment and health

Research has now moved on from establishing the link between unemployment and health to examining the nature of the relationship (Bartley 1994). She suggests four types of explanation for the effect of unemployment on health: poverty, stress, lifestyle and the long-term impact of periods of unemployment on an individual's working career as a whole. To these we should add a possible health selection effect. Such a selection effect argues that it is the unhealthy who become unemployed through loss of competence, rather than the unemployed who become ill through lack of work.

Large-scale cross sectional studies have revealed that a correlation between health and unemployment exists, but this category of study cannot give evidence of the direction of any causal link which is identified. For instance, evidence from the Longitudinal Survey shows that a health selection effect can only explain part of the increased mortality of the unemployed. Higher mortality was observed in those who had no apparent ill-health at the start of the study period. As well, the fact that unemployment affects the partners of the unemployed also seems to run counter to a selection effect explanation (Moser *et al.* 1990).

The British Regional Heart Study data also reveals that a selection effect cannot in itself explain the raised mortality of unemployed men. It has been tentatively argued that a causal link between unemployment and mortality can be identified (Morris *et al.* 1992). But they are less sure in isolating the mechanisms of this causal link. Amazingly, lifestyle factors (such as smoking) do not seem to explain the differences. Poverty, it is suggested, must be the mechanism by which unemployment affects health. Let us then consider poverty.

Following the publication of the Black Report (Townsend and Davidson 1982), the association between income and health inequalities has been much debated in Britain. Overwhelming is the weight of evidence which supports the view that inequalities based on social class exist. Blaxter (1990), drawing on the results of the Health and Lifestyle Survey, argues that the link between class and health is essentially a link between income and health. Blackburn (1991) advances three processes by which poverty could affect health: physiological, psychological and behaviour. The National Food Survey, cited by Blackburn, evokes the concerns of work of the 1930s, showing that a healthy diet costs more than an unhealthy one and may be beyond the reach of those reliant on state benefits. We can show that low income is likely to lead to poor housing, which is itself associated with reduced health outcomes (Best 1995). Trying to separate out different factors poses some difficulties. Wilson and Walker (1993), for example, argue that unemployment is often combined with other recognised social disadvantages: low social class, poor housing and poor local environment, all acting in concert.

The role of stress is familiar to anyone, from whatever social class, who has experienced unemployment. Empirically, it is clearly associated with raised levels of mental stress. Work does offer more than financial benefits to the employee, argues Jahoda (1982). Paid employment imposes a time structure on activity, it enlarges the circle of social interaction beyond the family circle, it provides participation in purposive group actions and imposes regular activity, among a host of other positive outcomes.

The hypothesis that the unemployed do not have access to the psychological benefits of paid work that Jahoda describes, but argues that denial of these benefits can explain only a minor part of the increased stress experienced by the unemployed, is supported by the work of Gershuny (1994). Fagin and Little's (1984) qualitative analysis of the experiences of the unemployed families does lend support to Jahoda's explanations of the negative effects of unemployment on psychological health. For instance, they found that the unemployed men had difficulty in structuring their days, and tasks that would previously have been completed in minutes could seem to stretch out for the whole day. Warr (1985) proposed nine mechanisms by which unemployment affects mental health. These mechanisms incorporate much of Jahoda's model but Warr argues that poverty is the factor likely to have the greatest single effect on psychological health. Unemployment brings loss of income and insecurity about meeting living expenses, and these factors themselves have psychosocial consequences.

Thus Warr showed that unemployment affects not only the quantity of interactions outside the home, but also their quality. Unemployment consistently leads to an increase in experiences which undermine the morale of the individual. Unsuccessful job applications, being regarded as a failure both by self and others, and the felt humiliation of being reliant on social security support, all must act to reduce self-esteem. On the other hand, Warr and Jackson (1985) were able to demonstrate that a return to employment brought about an improvement in psychological wellbeing, suggesting that unemployment was the initial causal factor.

Victim blaming

It is often easier to blame individuals than to suggest that social policy might be wrong. Accordingly, and not surprisingly, lifestyle explanations for ill-health have gained in currency in recent years. *The Health of the Nation* targets for health emphasise official concern to reduce perceived risk behaviours, such as smoking and drinking (DOH 1992). Evidence exists, of course, to suggest that unemployment leads to less healthy lifestyles. For one thing, the unemployed are likely to fall into other categories that are associated with 'unhealthy' behaviour patterns, such as low income and social class (Blaxter 1990).

Statistics show that the unemployed are heavier smokers, but this seems to reflect behaviour patterns that existed prior to unemployment (Morris, Cook and Shaper 1992). A review of the field by Cooper (1995) argues that it is difficult to conclude that unemployment is likely to lead to increased smoking and alcohol intake.

It is a regrettable fact that the effect of one spell of unemployment may carry on after a return to paid work. Thus, psychological effects of unemployment may extend well beyond the unemployed themselves to those who are in insecure employment. In that sense, unemployment should be seen as the extreme of a range of employment conditions in which job security is the key factor. People who have been unemployed once are more likely to take up insecure jobs and then experience subsequent unemployment (Burchell 1994).

Moreover, the risk of unemployment is not spread evenly through society. A relatively small section of society experiences the majority of unemployment (Bartley 1994).

Identifying the unemployed

While it can be concluded that there is a causal relationship between unemployment and health, it does not necessarily follow that all the unemployed experience poorer health outcomes. For some, the experience of unemployment can be positive in the same way that, for some, the experience of poverty can be positive (Smith 1987; Fagin and Little 1984). In health promotion it is important to identify those groups most at risk of the ill affects of unemployment. To perceive the unemployed as a conglomerate or underclass does not help the analysis. Gershuny and Marsh (1994) suggest that the attributes of a group who seem to have a proneness to unemployment should be recognised. We know that unemployment is not randomly distributed among the working population, the most significant predictor of a period of unemployment being a previous history of job loss. Worst affected are manual workers who form 75 per cent of the UK unemployed. Also young people are more likely to be unemployed. As well, both of these groups are more likely to become unemployed at some point, but are not necessarily likely to remain unemployed for longer periods (Layard *et al.* 1994).

The actual length of time spent without work is apparently crucial in its subsequent effects. The most intractable problems of unemployment are associated with long-term unemployment. In the UK 37 per cent of the total number of unemployed have been so for more than twelve months and more than 50 per cent have been unemployed for more than six months (Convery 1996). Obviously long-term unemployment compounds the effects of poverty, because savings get used up and the proportionate cost of renewing material goods increases.

In this way the long-term unemployed become trapped in a downward spiral of increasing disadvantage involving negative social class mobility, poorer health outcomes and loss of owner-occupied housing (Moser *et al.* 1987). Eventually, some studies suggest, some of the long-term unemployed 'adapt to their fate'. Psychological stress for the unemployed peaks after twelve to eighteen months, although high levels continue thereafter (Warr and Jackson 1985). There is some evidence that those who continue to expect to find work suffer more than those who become resigned to their position, possibly because the disappointment of continual failure is reinforced (Gallie and Vogler 1994).

Targeting health promotion at the unemployed

Any attempt to provide community support for the unemployed must take account of these economic, social, biomedical and political issues.

In 1987, Smith reported that a series of articles he had done on the health of the unemployed drew mixed reactions from the readership of the *British Medical Journal*. Some readers went so far go to argue that unemployment was a political and socio-economic issue, but not a medical one. This was rebuffed by Smith, who provided three counter arguments to this approach:

1 doctors should not be afraid of acting in an area where there is a clearly harmful effect on health;
2 doctors cannot choose but to be involved because they will have patients presenting with conditions associated with unemployment;
3 health workers are in a position to do something to alleviate the impact of unemployment.

However, it cannot be denied that there is an important point to be made about the efficacy of biomedicine in dealing with socially-based health issues. We are unsure of the precise biological mechanism by which unemployment affects health, but the reductionist science of biomedicine operates in other areas too at this level of ambiguity. In many respects, the situation is analogous to the reductions in death from infectious diseases which began before biomedicine discovered the biological basis for the conditions and their cures. Spectacular improvements come about due to social changes in living standards (Nettleton 1995). Hence, it is pertinent to question what the biomedical approach can now usefully contribute to improving the health status of the unemployed.

Through *The Health of the Nation* document, a way forward to improve the nation's health has been enshrined in government policy. The argument has been presented that health education has aimed to change the behaviour of individuals so as to encourage them to adopt healthier lifestyles. It has been said that the focus is on changing individuals to adapt to the environment rather than making the environment itself a healthier place in which to live. In that respect, health education can be seen as a form of 'victim blaming'; individuals are told that they can control their own health outcomes with the corollary that those who fail to do so are somehow responsible for their own failing. It is particularly easy to persuade many of the unemployed of this.

Clearly, any health education approach should take account of Jahoda and Warr's descriptions of the psychological effects of job loss. Individuals whose self-esteem is already undermined by the compounding effects of unemployment may not have the control over their behaviour that the individual, as

133

responsible actor model of health promotion, demands. Their level of empowerment is unlikely to be adequate to the task.

Thus, programmes that aim to alter individual behaviour may for these reasons be less successful among the unemployed. One significant study revealed that the unemployed find it harder to give up smoking, even though they may be well informed about the health risks involved, than do employed people (Lee *et al.* 1991).

Evidence from the Health and Lifestyles Survey seems to corroborate these concerns, questioning the efficacy of health education approaches aimed at altering behaviour patterns. Lifestyle factors are not as significant as social factors in explaining the worse health of low socio-economic groups, the survey shows. Likewise, moving away from perceived health risk behaviour does little to improve the health of the disadvantaged. In fact, the most significant factor affecting health at this level is social circumstance (Blaxter 1990). Disempowerment of the unemployed, in that health education may actual worsen the relative health of the poor as higher social groups show greater response to such behaviour change campaigns, is a possible outcome (Vagero 1991).

Publications consistently argue that health promotion involves social and environmental activities, which impinge on the ability of the individual to control their health outcomes and take appropriate action at local and national government level (WHO 1984). To that extent the practice of health promotion provides a stronger framework than either biomedicine or health education for addressing the causes of poor health among the unemployed. Obviously health promotion is a political activity and to try to deny the political as an appropriate sphere of action is in itself to adopt a political position supportive of the *status quo*. It is, of course, possible to accept the political nature of health work and still support a continuation of current policies, but the challenge presented by this appraisal is for health workers to be able to take up informed political positions. In the context of unemployment, this must involve understanding alternatives to the current orthodoxy that high unemployment is inevitable and recognising that socio-economic and political implications are two of these alternatives.

The first principle, that of defining what health is, has political connotations and the reader appreciates that biomedical models that describe health in terms of the presence or absence of disease have different implications for policy over more social models, such as that by the WHO. The WHO describes health as complete physical, mental and social wellbeing; consequently those who want paid employment but are without it would by this model be described as being unhealthy (Smith 1987).

In operational terms, health promotion has tended to attempt to address the effect of unemployment on health in two domains: that which seeks to alleviate the experience of unemployment and those that seek to reduce the overall number of unemployed. The Unemployment and Health Study Group

(1984) and Naidoo and Wills (1994) argue that health promoters and health-care providers are currently directed to work in the former domain, but it should not be forgotten that the theoretical basis of health promotion also' requires action in the latter. Let us consider these two separately.

Alleviation

The principal contributory factors to poor health in the unemployed are stress and poverty, and measures to alleviate the health impact of unemployment can be divided into those that address each of these.

The effects of stress

Jahoda's work indicates that the stresses of unemployment can only be relieved by a return to the paid employment role, while others have argued that some remedial action should be taken. The Unemployment and Health Study Group (1984) suggests that healthcare providers should be aware of the needs of the unemployed and plan the provision of services accordingly. Important in this respect is the provision of locally-based services, especially community mental health services. Social support networks can anticipate the stressful effects of unemployment, according to Wilson and Walker (1993). GPs are encouraged to be proactive in providing services for the unemployed.

But all such approaches call for effective targeting of resources. For instance, in areas of high unemployment, such as mining communities, where the main local employer has shut down, it may be easier to direct services appropriately, whereas the unemployed in communities where the majority of people are in work would be harder to target. However, people in this latter circumstance may be those in greatest need, for the stigma of unemployment is reduced when it becomes the norm within a community.

Poverty and the benefits system

Since 1930, poverty has been recognised as probably the main cause of health problems for the unemployed. Many commentators have concluded that attention should be paid to the benefit system to ensure that benefits are paid at a rate that prevents poverty effects (Smith 1987; Wilson and Walker 1993). A simple solution is to raise the level of benefits. However, in practice, former government policy has been the reverse; namely, to reduce benefits, thus increasing the relative poverty of the unemployed.

Health promoters need to be aware of the political and economic debate that surrounds the level of state benefits. For some, the existence of benefits acts as a disincentive to find new jobs, and the higher the level of benefit, the less likely that people will seek work.

However, Nimmo (1996) challenges the popular belief that benefits create a culture of dependency in which the recipients lose motivation to seek work. He shows that the long-term unemployed are characterised, not so much as in having lost the motivation to find work, but in lacking the skills and resources required by the job market. Similar conclusions are reached by Gallie and Vogler (1994), namely, it is not lack of motivation but lack of opportunity that distinguishes the long-term unemployed. At a wider level, the political consequences of raising benefits is clear – the threat of a rise in taxation – and that, rather than any academic analysis of the problem, is doubtless the reason for lack of action.

Reduction of unemployment

Economists debate whether high levels of unemployment are avoidable. Indeed, the then Chancellor, Norman Lamont, memorably argued in 1991 that unemployment was a price worth paying to reduce inflation (Clark and Layard 1993). Note that there was little likelihood of him paying the price!

Other economists do question the view that there is an inevitable trade-off between unemployment and inflation (Layard et al. 1994). All sorts of telling economic arguments can be made that unemployment is not an inevitable fact of economic life, but now it is widely accepted that the reality is that high levels of unemployment can be expected to continue for the foreseeable future (Bartley 1994).

Layard et al. (1994) demonstrate that long-term unemployment is highest in those European countries which pay benefits for an indefinite period. This stands in stark contrast to the USA, where payments cease after six months or with Sweden where fourteen months is the maximum. There are differences, though. The Swedish model is associated with strong labour market prices designed to find people productive work. These embrace proactive employment exchange workers, high-quality retraining services aimed at providing the skills required by the employment market, recruitment incentives for employers and the right to temporary public employment in the last resort. Throughout the 1980s, the Swedish model was successful in keeping unemployment rates low in comparison to the rest of Europe, and in eliminating the problem of long-term unemployment. Such an approach appears expensive to the tax-payer, but is effectively self-financing when the overall savings of reduced unemployment benefit payments are considered.

Benzeval et al. (1995) conclude that any strategy to reduce health inequalities must include measures to reduce unemployment to the lowest possible level. Four recent efforts to formulate policies geared to the reduction of unemployment were identified by them. Common themes included: an emphasis on education and training, changes to the benefit and taxation system, the promotion of new patterns of work and encouraging entrepreneurship. Encouragement of such policies is presented as a proper focus of health promotion. It is not within the scope of this chapter to rehearse all of the different economic arguments, only to assert that health promoters need to be involved in the debates. The Swedish benefits model presented above serves as an example that alternative approaches to perceived political orthodoxy do exist.

Health promotion provides a focus of convergence, by which these can be discussed collectively from a health perspective. Alternative approaches based on biomedicine or health education cannot alone hope to address the health issues raised by unemployment. Of course, this does involve claiming the socio-economic and the political, as well as the individual, as the appropriate spheres of activity of health promotion.

Health promotion targeted at the employed

On the coat-tails of the 'smoking makes you sick' awareness, many larger businesses in the USA realised that it made sound commercial sense to encourage employees to adopt a healthy lifestyle, even if doing so involved financial outlay. Accordingly, by the mid-1970s, an increasing number of American corporations and businesses had introduced health promotion or 'wellness' programmes into the workplace. Such programmes 'differ from the traditional occupational health mission in that wellness programmes are interested in general health promotion among employees, rather than focusing on health protection, i.e. preventing occupational diseases or ensuring safe working conditions' suggests Conrad (1988). The orientation of these programmes, then, is to facilitate changing people's behaviour or lifestyle in order to prevent disease and to promote health.

Since 1978, the emergence of the 'lifestyle risk factor' paradigm has refocused the direction of public health issues and health promotion in particular. Slowly but inexorably, the realisation by the general public that lifestyle behaviours, such as smoking, exercise habits and dietary factors, predispose synergistically to the modern 'diseases of affluence' – cardiovascular disease and malignancies – has attained currency. This has led to a shift from the assumption that health depended on control of disease, and therefore on medical intervention by physicians, toward a view which gave more emphasis to individual responsibility. Instead, it has become clear that there are no miracle cures for the new killers and that they are largely the result of the lifestyle of the individual. We now know that, exactly as illness is caused by identifiable factors, health is likewise so mediated, the relevant factors being determined by nutrition, physical fitness, handling of stress, choice of environment and use of alcohol, tobacco and drugs. In short, they are controlled by behaviour and can be controlled only by its modification.

In the USA this became abundantly obvious and is perhaps best illustrated by the move to a healthier lifestyle in which jogging became a national pastime, health-food stores mushroomed and people switched from eating high-cholesterol animal fats to cholesterol-free vegetable oils, resulting in a striking decrease in death from coronary heart disease between 1968 and 1977, a 22 per cent decline (Farquhar 1978). Indubitably, the change from unhealthy behaviours and lifestyles began with the motivation of individuals to assume more personal responsibility for their health. Fitness programmes, tended to provide education and a supportive environment necessary for monitoring a change in lifestyle. Individuals were aided to identify health risks, and then instruction was given to modify behaviour so as to eliminate those risks to health. Additionally, these programmes introduced the individual to the concept of wellness. However, this trend towards lifestyle intervention at a personal level must be balanced against the knowledge that individuals may not have the desire, control or ability to make lifestyle changes. Some commentators, such as Conrad (1988), warn of the 'dangers of overstating individual responsibility for health and the dangers of crossing the thin line to blaming the victim'. In this we confront again the concept of empowerment.

In many respects, the workplace is an ideal starting venue for intervention with a largely captive audience and the capability of influencing behaviour through the rules and regulations of the organisation, the provision of facilities and the working conditions of the employees. After all, workers spend more than 30 per cent of their waking hours at work so the workplace should have enormous potential for mediating health education and promotion. As Conrad points out:

> Corporate executives and managers are attracted by the broad claims made for worksite health promotion which include : improving employees' health and fitness; decreasing medical and disability costs; reducing absenteeism; decreasing turnover; improving employee mental alertness, moral and job satisfaction; increasing productivity; and enhancing the corporate image.
>
> (Conrad 1988)

Determinants of the extent of health promotion provision

Privatised healthcare, especially the system in the USA, became the catalyst which focused attention on the ideology of workplace health promotion. By the late 1970s several large employers there discovered that their corporate health insurance premiums were consistently outpacing inflation. It was this realisation, together with a growing body of evidence to suggest that company healthcare costs are strongly related to employee lifestyle and behaviour patterns, that served to galvanise the employers into addressing the issue. Establishment of the link between medical claims for conditions largely attributable to lifestyle factors led to an acknowledgement that behaviour-related improvements in health should lead to containment of costs. In response to this, workplace health promotion programmes have flourished.

Naturally, given the complexity of the statistics involved, the data concerning the relationship between employee health and economic benefits is not yet conclusive (as many of the programmes have been in existence for a relatively short period of time), but the initial success demonstrated by companies like Du Pont and Johnson & Johnson have ensured that workplace health promotion has now become a corporate norm in the USA. Recent surveys, including the US Department of Health and Human Services' (1985) national survey of worksite health promotion activities, have amply confirmed this fact. The survey revealed that of 1,358 companies employing fifty or more staff, 65.8 per cent had some form of workplace health promotion activity and more that half of these had been running for over five years (Penack 1991). There are many examples, such as the study in 1987 by the Heart Research Institute, which demonstrated that 63 per cent of respondents from Fortune's 500 largest industrial corporations offered health promotion activities of one kind or another. Most frequently the programmes offered emphasised weight reduction and smoking cessation, followed by fitness and stress reduction programmes (Hollander and Largerman 1988). In Britain, as employers increasingly offer private health insurance schemes to a wide range of employees, the economic benefits of workplace health promotion programmes experiences in North America are becoming more relevant on the UK scene.

> Given that the American programmes have been tailored to the different circumstances of the employees and organisations in question, there is no reason to believe that programmes in the UK, likewise tailored to the staff and organisations, would not yield comparably positive results.
>
> (Bovell 1992)

Consider the following figures. In 1986, the Health Education Authority surveyed eighty-five organisations, gaining a response from 50 per cent. More than half of Britain's workers had no access to basic occupational health services then, but there was growing recognition of the role of the workplace in health promotion. Such health promotion programmes had tended to be adopted on an *ad hoc* basis, rather than as a specific policy for health promotion, with only episodic evaluation of the effectiveness of programmes (Jacobson *et al.* 1988).

But again, in 1991, the extent and nature of the provision of employee health and welfare programmes in a range of private and public sector organisations was surveyed (Watson 1992). A postal questionnaire to 300 organisations, with a 50 per cent response rate, revealed that around half of respondents had provided health promotion programmes, with higher rates of provision in private sector and health authorities compared to local authorities. Three principal categories of health promotion programme were extant:

1   Problem-centred programmes, directly involving individuals on a one-to-one basis, such as counselling for work and non-work problems, e.g. the use and abuse of alcohol.
2   Programmes aimed at changing and supporting the change of individual lifestyles, involving both policy implementation and the introduction of initiatives to support policies, such as providing a non-smoking policy and providing initiatives to help smokers stop smoking.
3   Programmes aimed at secondary prevention, such as the early detection of diseases through screening. These involved a much heavier emphasis on theoretical education.

Even more recently the Health Education Authority (HEA) surveyed a sample of 1,344 workplaces in England (HEA 1993) and this showed that health promotion in the workplace was seen to be a very important issue by 69 per cent of very large workplaces, but only by 41 per cent of small workplaces. This relationship between large and small business also hold true for smoking, with 81 per cent of large companies with more than 500 employees having smoking-related activities, compared to only 31 per cent of small companies. Smoking was considered to be the most important health-related activity, but health promotion activities are quite varied, ranging from general screening policies to strategies on blood control (see Table 1).

Table 1   Range of activities by size of workplace (unweighted base: 1344)

	Number of employees (%)				
Activity	*All workplaces*	*1–24*	*25–99*	*100–499*	*500+*
Smoking	31	30	44	64	81
Alcohol	14	14	21	31	46
Health eating	6	5	14	29	47
Catering	5	4	15	33	45
Stress	8	8	13	19	32
HIV/AIDS	9	8	16	26	42
Weight control	3	3	5	16	30
Exercise/fitness	6	6	12	22	37
Heart health	4	3	8	22	43
Breast screening	3	2	5	16	29
Cervical screening	3	3	5	14	23
General screening	5	4	11	32	54
Lifestyle assessment	3	3	2	6	21
Cholesterol testing	4	4	5	13	24
Blood pressure control	4	3	8	19	44
Drugs/substance abuse	5	5	12	15	28

Altogether, these findings may be seen as moderately encouraging, but must be interpreted with caution (Sanders 1993). For instance, the degree of reported health promotion activity may be an over-estimate of the true extent of activity, due to response bias. Companies with an interest in health promotion may be more likely to respond to surveys than those with little interest and little or no activity, giving a much higher estimated rate of health promotion in the UK workplace. Reviewing the literature on the extent of health promotion at work in the UK, Philo and Freedman (1992) conclude that, compared with other countries, there is a very low rate of workplace health initiatives in the UK. In the UK there is no legal requirement for occupational health services, other than in exceptionally dangerous occupations, and there is very little development of a co-ordinated occupational health service in the NHS (Harvey 1988). Nevertheless, there is some cause for optimism as highlighted in *The Health of the Nation*:

Employers have long been required to provide safe working conditions. Increasingly they are also recognising the benefits of a healthy workforce, while trade unions and staff associations are looking for more ways to improve the general health of their membership.

(DOH 1992)

Changing attitudes to employment and health

In some senses, as Tones (1990) argues, the relationship between work and health is paradoxical. 'On the one hand those of a Marxist persuasion may view work as a capitalist device to exploit the proletariat' whereas on the other hand 'a more common stand-point is that unemployment rather than work is health damaging'. The same writers comment further that 'the more conventional analysis of work and health sees the workplace as a source of pathogens of one kind or another, ranging from general work-produced stress to specific industrial hazards such as accidents, cancer and the like'.

That there indeed is a link between an individual's health in the broadest sense, and the nature of his/her work, is now increasingly accepted. Twenty years ago and more it was known that, in Britain, rates of sickness absence were found to have been rising continuously in the 1960s (Taylor 1974). Such a rise is difficult to explain in purely epidemiological terms since, during the same period, there was a decline in the number of days lost through diseases such as TB, pneumonia and stomach/duodenal ulcers, which had traditionally produced a significant volume of sickness absence. On the other hand, other causes such as 'sprains and strains', 'nerves, debility and headache' and psychoneurosis have increased (Taylor 1974). That is, 'harder', more objectively identifiable causes of sickness absence have been replaced by more subjective psychosomatic ones, and it is this phenomenon which needs to be explained. As Jenny Lisle (1993) points out:

There is increasing evidence that an unsatisfactory work environment may lead to psychological disorders. Studies have shown that contributory factors are work overload, lack of control over one's work, limited job opportunities, role ambiguity and conflict, non-supportive supervisors or co-workers and machine paced work.

In recent years such factors have been linked to chronic 'stress' disorders. This means that attempts to explain present trends in sickness absence more fully must, therefore, take into account the more qualitative aspects of work and of the working environment. Failure of top management to attend to these organisational stressors may undercut any well-intended efforts, aimed at the individual to reduce stress through health promotion programmes.

But, as health promoters are fully aware, it is not just stress at work that can lead to ill-health. An entire matrix of mechanisms whereby work affects health are numerous and far reaching. Four key areas were identified by Harvey (1988), as follows:

1   Income – by determining an individual's (or family unit's) ability to pay for goods and service. Health status also affects their ability to work and earn.
2   Work environment – the quality of the environment and the work processes may affect workers' health. The direct results are seen in accidents and occupational diseases. Working conditions can also be contributory factors in morbidity and mortality, such as heart disease and lung cancer.
3   Work outputs – consumable goods, services and waste by-products affect both the health of workers and that of the wider population and environments.
4   Mental health – work involves psychological costs and benefits.

According to a report from an Independent Multidisciplinary Committee (Ashton and Gill 1991), only a small proportion of the total mortality resulting from exposure to occupational health hazards is currently identifiable. As the Committee points out 'even what should be regarded as an occupational risk becomes hard to define. For instance, if exercise is beneficial to health, should the increasing tendency to sedentary work be regarded as an occupational hazard?'

Members of the committee go on to suggest that one way of establishing the influence of occupation on mortality is to assume social class is a good guide to the health risks associated with people's domestic circumstances and way of life. That would allow us to compare the variation on death rates between occupations before and after standardising them for their social class. Using twenty-five occupational categories and six social classes, one study showed that 80 per cent of the mortality variation seemed to be associated with 'way of life' (i.e. social class) and the rest with occupation (Fox and Adelstein 1978).

Is employee health promotion worth it?

It is now obvious that corporate organisations have a unique opportunity to exert a major, perhaps even a decisive, effect on the health of the population in the third millennium. Indeed the incentive for companies and organisations to act has never been greater. It has been established by the Confederation of British Industry that absenteeism costs Britain in excess of £5 billion per year (Bovell 1992). David Ashton (1989) asserts: 'A corporate NHS focused on the prevention of disease and the promotion of health in the workplace, is not only medically desirable but also commercially and economically sensible'.

Large-scale organisations are fond of claiming that the most important asset they possess is their workforce, so much so that the saying 'people are our most important asset' has become one of the modern-day corporate mantras. If that is true, therefore, then all corporate organisations should be interested in the health of their employees. It is not difficult to isolate other, more specific, reasons:

1   Health promotion and other strategies of preventive medicine in the workplace are not only a means of improving the health of the workforce. They can also constitute a powerful vehicle by which to enhance the company image and to establish goodwill with the local community.
2   In order to bring about permanent changes in behaviour, it is necessary to create an atmosphere and a culture which is supportive of the kind of behaviour change one is trying to bring about. For example, a heavy cigarette smoker will find it infinitely more difficult to give up in an environment where smoking is permitted than in one in which a smoking policy is properly in force and the culture is broadly supportive.

All such initiatives cost money and the question remains as to what companies or organisations can reasonably expect in return for their efforts? Evidence has unambiguously shown that there is a clear relationship between the health and wellbeing of the workforce and their productivity. For example, Kimberly-Clark executives in the US believe that the company's health promotion programme has enabled them to recruit higher calibre employees and to reduce absenteeism (Ashton 1989; Penack 1991; Dedman 1986). In the same way, Du Pont (also in the USA) were able to demonstrate a 47.5 per cent decline in hourly absenteeism over six years, in a site participating in their workplace health promotion programme, compared to a 12.5 per cent decline in the total Du Pont hourly workforce (Bertera 1991). A whole litany of consequences springs from this and we see a strong connection between worksite health promotion programmes and reduced absenteeism rates, reduced accident rates, improved productivity, reduced health insurance claims and, in the longer term, reduced illness, premature disability and death.

In the US context, Bovell (1992) has reviewed the literature on the cost-effectiveness of workplace health promotion programmes. He concludes that benefits have been seen in a number of areas, such as:

Absences from work The evidence suggests that those workplace health promotion interventions that are systematically organised, available to all staff, well-resourced, supported by management and continue for some time, lead to significant reductions in the overall level of absence from work. Falls in absenteeism of between 9 per cent and 29 per cent have been reported, with an increase in absence rates in control groups not subject to health promotion intervention.

Productivity An overview of the research indicates that health promotion in the workplace can lead to a 4 per cent gain in productivity.

Staff attitude and morale Health promotion programmes are associated with improvements in morale, assessed by measures such as attitudes towards the organisation and staff relations.

Staff turnover Following the introduction of health promotion prog-rammes, staff turnover is reduced.

Less tangible benefits, such as improved morale and improved employer–employee relations, are more difficult to quantify but are no less important. There is even strong evidence suggesting that such programmes have a high perceived value among the workforce and can do much to create and to maintain good working attitudes.

Since in recent years we have been asked to contemplate the idea of a 'corporate NHS', it is interesting to note that the Secretary of State, as part of the national strategy for health, has recently launched a new initiative entitled 'Health at Work in the NHS'. In the long term, this project aims to: 'Introduce a systematic healthy workplace programme throughout the NHS; and engage all NHS staff in health promoting activities'.

The hope and expectation is that this will result in the NHS becoming an exemplary employer over the next ten years, demonstrating to others that a healthy workhorse benefits both individual staff members and the organisa-tion as a whole. According to the Health at Work in the NHS Pack, the intention is 'to include all NHS workplaces, such as hospitals, clinics, admin-istrative headquarters, ambulance stations, GP surgeries and health centres. Staff residences will not be overlooked'.

Impact on the British population of workplace health promotion

In Britain, the workplace offers access to 26 million adults (Jacobson *et al.* 1991), the majority of whom are young and often difficult to reach through other means. For example, people of working age are the most infrequent attendees at GP surgeries (Stoute 1989). The context of employment offers several types of approach for health promotion and disease prevention. Moreover, as a major proportion of the workforce are manual workers, there are also special opportunities to reach many of the people who are most at risk, not only of work-related ill-health, but of many other aspects of ill-health. Jacobson *et al.* (1988) suggest five categories of approach based on the main health hazards being targeted:

1   hazards found in the workplace that can be the direct cause of injury or disability;
2   hazards at work which can be contributory causes of disease;
3   hazards at work which can aggravate existing disease or latent conditions;
4   situations in which work offers easy access to potential hazards;
5   areas in which the health of the employees can be influenced by health promotion programmes at work, and in which there can be significant benefits to employers from tackling such issues.

We have seen, then, that the literature on health promotion at work is characterised by a general shift in focus from hazard-reduction to health promotion (Philo and Freedman 1992) and emphasises individual behaviour and lifestyles, to the exclusion of environmental and organisational factors. But, as the rest of this book makes clear, the individual lifestyle approach (which in some instances may be perceived as 'victim blaming') is only one part of the picture. To give a cogent example, teaching individuals how to manage stress is only of limited value if one does not also address the organisational causes of stress.

12

HEALTH PROMOTION AND TOBACCO USE

Why tobacco use is different

With reference to alcohol, one would legitimately refer to its 'use' and 'abuse', although, in the latter category, it is the drinker rather than the alcohol which becomes abused. However, when it comes to tobacco, agreement is virtually unanimous in holding that any use of it for human consumption constitutes an abuse of health. It is the very strength of this assurance that so strongly differentiates the complementary roles of health education and health promotion. Indeed, the links between tobacco use and ill-health have been so strongly established, and continue to become even more strongly established with almost every piece of published research in the area, that the health education task is overwhelmingly simple. What is less readily appreciated is the extent to which this may not only be irrelevant in the struggle of many people in their daily lives for health, but may actually further disempower them.

It has been well established that people do not smoke through ignorance of its adverse effects on health. They rarely even begin to take up a smoking lifestyle in their early teens due to such ignorance. When this author meets people living on Income Support, as close to the edge of economic ruin as one can get, a sentiment often shared with him is that 'without my fags, I couldn't get on'. In other words, in their experience, health (as meaning one's capacity to go on from day to day) involves larger concerns than clinical or physiological 'wellness'. Again, one frequently hears from secondary school students that they know very well that smoking is dangerous and that by smoking they are only making money for some large corporation that 'doesn't care a toss' for them. They understand that perfectly well. But they still smoke because it resolves many more immediately pressing social and psychological problems for them.

Therefore, for health promotion to confront tobacco use, it has to be aware of the following:

1   Tobacco use presents two immediate problems each with a different set of resolution strategies:

    a   how to impact cognitively on non-smokers in such a way that they realise empowerment by not starting;
    b   how to bring smokers to the point at which they find that quitting is more self-enhancing than is continuing.

2   Conventional health education, with its well-referenced and thoroughly rational, scientific arguments against tobacco use by people, can serve to undermine empowerment and render attempts at health promotion counter-productive.

In this chapter, we shall concentrate on the role of health promotion in smoking cessation programmes, especially, but not exclusively, in the context of primary health care. Of course, there are many areas in which smoking behaviour and health promotion interact, but in the primary health care setting we have the one most likely to be visited by people on a reasonably regular basis and not necessarily for reasons to do with tobacco use. It therefore affords, probably, the greatest single scope for the application of health promotion to the problem.

In primary health care the focus on health promotion results from a diversity of influences. Changing patterns of disease and the accompanying emphasis on preventive health, combined with changes in health care policy, provision, and practice, have influenced and delineated the practitioner's role and performance within health promotion programmes. Consistent with these changes, there has been an increase in research from within the medical and nursing professions, to discover the most effective way to achieve a healthy lifestyle within a population. Research concerning smoking cessation and optimum behaviour change has burgeoned recently and should influence health promotion initiatives directed at smoking cessation programmes run within the primary healthcare setting.

Obviously, social and psychological influences upon smoking behaviour can also affect the efficacy of any planned smoking cessation programmes. Therefore, these factors, combined with those already mentioned, highlight the need for effective monitoring and evaluation methods in health promotion.

Health promotion in the context of primary health

The Royal College of General Practitioners, in its paper 'Prevention of Arterial Disease in General Practice' in 1981, declared it imperative that primary healthcare teams have a greater involvement in activities aimed at preventing coronary heart disease. General Practitioners (GPs) were

147

encouraged to assume a greater responsibility for providing health education and this would involve giving advice on smoking, diet and alcohol, as well as routinely including specific screening procedures for hypertension and serum cholesterol. Research by Fullard and her colleagues in Oxford (1984) lent credence to this enterprise and it led to the introduction of the 'health check' as a popular form of preventive care within the general practice setting. Ordinarily these checks were carried out by practice nurses, rather than the doctor and involved the measurement of blood pressure, height and weight and the provision of advice on smoking reduction and other aspects of cardiovascular risk.

Such an approach to community healthcare was consistent with the wider changes introduced in the Government White Paper on primary care, *Promoting Better Health* (DHSS 1987). This document affirmed the Government's commitment to a change of emphasis from treatment to prevention and it encouraged family doctors and primary healthcare teams to 'increase their contribution to the promotion of good health' (DHSS 1987).

The White Paper was primarily concerned with the development of health promotion and the prevention of ill-health by the explicit application of health education within primary care. It strongly urged the establishment of more health promotion sessions in general practice, in which advice on how to give up smoking was a key feature, in addition to the provision of regular and frequent health checks. As an incentive to achieve this outcome, doctors were to be offered financial incentives for the number of health checks performed and screening targets achieved. The consequent increase in health promotion activity and the removal of restrictions on the number and type of staff whom the doctors could employ through the direct reimbursement scheme, both led to an increase in the number of practice nurses employed and Fullard *et al.* (1987) believe that these developments assured a role for the practice nurse in primary healthcare. Stilwell (1991) and Fry (1991) confirm this and have indeed established that most of the health promotion work within general practice is now carried out by practice nurses, rather than by other practice staff or the GP.

A subsequent document, *Working for Patients* (DHSS 1989), aimed to provide patients with better healthcare and greater choice and to reward those working in the NHS who were willing to respond specifically to local need. This approach finally recognised the effect of social and cultural differences upon health. However, the most significant change for primary healthcare was the introduction of GP fund holding and the notion that GP remuneration would be linked more directly to their level of performance.

All of this represented a sea-change in the culture of the old NHS and Hughes (1993) refers to these changes as 'the most radical reforms to funding and organisation of general medical practice since the Pilkington Commission in 1960'. As of 1990, the GP contract introduced target levels for: vaccination, immunisation, and cervical cancer screening, and remuneration for health promotion sessions in general practice. It also demanded the provision of regular health checks for particular sections of the community. Financial incentives were given as an inducement to GPs to undertake these new tasks. Hughes (1993) argued that the Government of the day regarded general practice as a cost-effective form of healthcare but he did question whether the subsequent response to the contract offered the most efficient preventive care or the best value for money, even then.

Research has been unanimous in confirming that target payments and sessional fees as a means of achieving policy objectives do work and they have been shown by Hughes and Yule (1993) to affect doctors' practice. However, what is not at all evident is whether the incentives serve to provide extra services or just to reorganise existing ones as a means of obtaining a sessional payment for providing them (Hughes 1993).

It was not long before such doubts prompted a further modification in that the lump sum fee, which had been payable to general practitioners who provided 'health promotion' clinics, was replaced by the new contracts introduced on 1 July 1993. A significant shift in emphasis, whereby GPs receive an annual lump sum payment to provide specific programmes of health promotion activity, was implicit in this new contract. Practices are now required to compile a minimum amount of information about a target percentage of the population and they are paid according to a banding system which is dependent upon the indicated intensity of intervention. Thus, the recording of smoking status and the provision of smoking cessation advice is a requirement of all bands and confirms smoking cessation as a key target for primary healthcare teams.

Morbidity and tobacco use

Tobacco has been smoked, chewed and sniffed, for centuries, and although the idea that its ingestion might cause cancer was first expressed by Sommering (1795) in Germany (cited in International Agency for Research on Cancer (IARC) 1986), only slight attention was paid to this until 1950, when several case control studies by Doll and Hill (1958) concluded that there was a clear association between smoking and lung cancer. Only a short while later, a further cohort study by them demonstrated an association between smoking and cancer of the lungs, respiratory and digestive tract; chronic bronchitis; coronary artery disease; peptic ulcer and cirrhosis of the liver (Doll and Hill 1964).

Cohort studies, as a statistical innovation, arose largely in the context of research on smoking and the most convincing of such studies to be carried out, which demonstrated the importance of smoking in the causation of cardiovascular disease, took place in the USA. A long-term follow-up study of a sample of adults from Framingham, in the state of Massachusetts, was begun in 1948. It considered factors such as blood cholesterol levels, blood pressure, cigarette smoking and body mass index and clearly heart disease (Shurtleff 1974).

There is clear and overwhelming evidence of the harmful effects of smoking, but despite this a comparatively high percentage of the population still smoke and there has been only a minimal change in smoking habits. During the early 1960s there was a decline in the total weight of tobacco sold as manufactured cigarettes, which may in part be due to the introduction of filters (Wald and Nicolaides-Bouman 1991), but the major decline in cigarette consumption was not experienced until the mid-1970s. It then continued to fall by 25 per cent over the following ten years (Wald and Nicolaides-Bouman 1991). But after that it seemed to level off and, since the mid-1980s there has been little change in the number of manufactured cigarettes sold (Tobacco Advisory Council; cited in Wald and Nicolaides-Bouman 1991).

The Office of Population and Census Surveys (OPCS) analysis in 1990, using findings from 1972 to 1988, showed that there was a decline in smoking among men from 52 per cent to 33 per cent, whereas among women it was less significant, from 41 per cent to 30 per cent. Parallel with this, there was a rise in the number of men who never or only occasionally smoked cigarettes from 25 per cent to 35 per cent, while there was a much smaller relative increase in such women from 49 per cent to 51 per cent.

Prior to the very extensive publicity about the harmful effects of smoking, there had been only a slight difference between the smoking habits of the different social classes in Britain. However, now the difference is marked, with a prevalence of 43 per cent of manual workers compared to 16 per cent among professional workers. Moreover, Whitehead (1987) has convincingly demonstrated that this difference is reflected in mortality rates. Thus, an unskilled man in social class five is three times more likely to die of lung cancer, and 25 per cent more likely to die of ischaemic heart disease, than is a man in social class one.

Sad to say, adolescents continue to take up cigarette smoking, especially in the last two years of school. Dobbs and Marsh (1983) established that 7 per cent of 13-year-olds smoked regularly and that the proportion rose to 26 per cent among 16-year-olds. They also ascertained that during the adolescent period, when smoking patterns are believed to be established, it was women who were more likely to emerge as smokers.

Each year in England and Wales it is estimated that there are 111,000 premature deaths and 284,000 hospital admissions caused by smoking, all of which adds an annual cost of £400 million to the NHS (DHSS 1993). It is no exaggeration to claim, therefore, that a Government strategy which addresses smoking as a key target area for action seems long overdue. *The Health of the Nation* (DOH 1992) does aim to reduce the prevalence of smoking in men and women over the age of sixteen to no more than 29 per cent by the year 2000.

General practice led smoking cessation programmes

The Health of the Nation (1992) adumbrates the proactive role that GPs and primary healthcare teams can play in achieving the targets for smoking. It asserts that GPs will be 'encouraged to record quantified information on patient smoking habits, for practice profiles, and it urges health professionals to give a higher priority to offering smoking cessation advice and support. Also it seeks to increase the numbers of patients visiting their GPs and who subsequently receive smoking cessation advice.

For a variety of reasons, it has gradually become evident that a number of factors render the general practice a suitable setting for preventive activities. Without doubt, the main one is that of access and opportunity. It has been established by Russell *et al.* (1979) that over 90 per cent of adults visit their GP at least once every five years, the average attendance exceeding three a year, and that smokers attend more often than non-smokers. In that way doctors have contact with a potentially high number of smokers and Ockene (1987) feels they are in an ideal situation to advise their patients on smoking cessation. The doctors are also the most likely member of the primary healthcare team to be in a position to present their patient with objective evidence of ill-health at the very time when the patient is most likely to be persuaded and to be especially vulnerable to the stop smoking message (Ahmed and Hilton 1982; Richmond and Webster 1985).

It has also been argued by Fowler (1993) that doctors are a 'good role model', as only 5 per cent of a random sample of British GPs were found to be cigarette smokers and anti-smoking advice, delivered by someone who models the principles advocated, has been found to be a highly credible source of influence (Lichtenstein *et al.* 1981). In addition, the GP consultation also offers a continuity of contact and an increased opportunity for face-to-face advice and counselling, which Sanders (1992) has shown to be more effective in changing people's behaviour.

At the level of rigorous analysis, there have been numerous randomised trials directed at evaluating the effects of a variety of GP administered smoking cessation programmes. Nevertheless, Heather (1989) and Sanders (1992) have found that any direct comparison of these studies is difficult, owing to the wide range of methodological differences. These include: different follow-up intervals, different criteria for abstinence, the extent to which self-reports of quitting were validated by bio-chemical measures, different methods of estimating abstinence rates and the criteria for entry to the trial. One serious problem, from an analytical stand-point, is that there has been no standardisation of interventions. For example, in situations which demand 'brief advice' as part of the intervention (Russell *et al.* 1979; Stewart and Rosser 1982), the extent and nature of the intervention is neither stated nor standardised. Major flaws like this notwithstanding, the majority of the studies do show that, generally, greater investment of GP time does produce higher abstention rates. But there have been a few notable exceptions. The analyses carried out by Stewart and Rosser (1982), Russell and Stapleton (1987) and Slama and Redman (1990) failed to find any long-term superiority between GP's brief advice over non-intervention and other control conditions. It has been pointed out that this may be due to the length and obtrusive nature of any extended behaviour change attempted (Slama and Redman 1990) which might have made the doctor less motivated to adhere to the programme or even to the mode of intervention altogether (Russell and Stapleton 1987; Stewart and Rosser 1982).

Very large studies by Russell et al. (1979), Russell and Stapleton (1983) and Jamrozik et al. (1984) have shown that, in a sample of more than 2,000 patients, brief advice from a doctor during a consultation can be effective in helping a small, but significant, number of patients to stop smoking. They have also shown, however, that higher cessation rates can occur with more intense intervention and increased contact from the physician. The maximum intervention in the initial research by Russell et al. (1979) consisted of advice, a leaflet and a follow-up appointment, whereas the more recent studies have dealt with interventions which included nicotine gum (Russell and Stapleton 1983) or carbon monoxide measurement (Jamrozik et al. 1984) in their programme.

In Australia two studies, carried out by Richmond and Webster (1985) and by Richmond et al. (1988) respectively, achieved an extremely high success rate. The 1985 study had a 33 per cent success rate after six months, following doctor advice and blood and lung function tests. This compared to a rate of 8 per cent in the control group. The 1986 study established that, of the thirty-seven patients who attended the entire programme and attended all follow-up visits, 57 per cent were abstinent at three years. These findings would seem to indicate that by personalising the effects of smoking by giving test results, chances of a successful outcomes are enhanced and that the use of nicotine gum and other self-help materials were useful additions to the GP's advice.

By contrast, these results may appear to compare badly with the English-based studies of Russell et al. (1979, 1988), Russell and Stapleton (1983) and Jamrozik et al. (1984), where the high intervention groups achieved a success rate of 5.1 per cent to 17 per cent. However, as Sanders (1992) argues, it is impossible to draw any definite conclusions about the relative effectiveness of specific interventions because of the methodological differences between the studies and the significant differences in sample size.

Employing meta-analysis of thirty-nine controlled triangles, Kottke (1988) attempted to discover if some characteristics other than the primary intervention itself might be the determinant of a successful intervention effect. One hundred and eight intervention comparisons were examined and the findings are eminently interesting, for they state that successful intervention is associated with personalised smoking advice and with assistance repeated in different forms and by several sources over the longest feasible period. That is, the overall recommendation from this analysis is that the message should be delivered 'clearly, repeatedly and consistently through every feasible delivery system' (Kottke 1988). It was also established that, with appropriate adjustment, the figures showed that the number of intervention modalities alone had a positive association with intervention success.

Clearly, increased intervention inevitably involves more time spent in consultation and greater effort at increased cost. Such resource intensive commitments, as required in these doctor-led programmes, may not seem to justify the outcome (Slama and Redman 1990). However, Ockene (1987) argues that it is worth the outlay as the relatively low cessation effect, coupled with the high contact, does have the potential to produce 'a high yield of ex-smokers' and consequently the physician-delivered smoking intervention could have 'a stronger impact on the health of patients than any other single intervention carried out in an out-patient setting'.

The evidence from these studies demonstrates that doctor intervention can be effective in stopping a small percentage of their patients smoking. However, there are other variables that may have an effect on outcome and we shall now consider two major ones.

First, consider the fact that the patients' own characteristics may influence the individual's chances of success (Lennox 1992), and in the study by Gilpin et al. (1992) smoking advice was found to be biased towards white middle-class groups. It is evident that this could have implications for GP practices with specific demographic and soci-economic features, in which targets are set for smoking as part of the normal GP contract. We know that attendance for primary healthcare also depends upon the motivation and attitude of the individual. It has also been found that it was those patients with the recognised risk factors, and who would potentially benefit most from health promotion, who were the least likely to attend for preventive healthcare; so fulfilling Hart's Inverse Care Law.

Tudor Hart (1971) made the provocative observation in a *Lancet* article to the effect that good healthcare tends to vary inversely with the need of the population. This is now referred to, especially in health promotion circles, as Hart's Inverse Care Law. What he meant by it, basically, was just because a health service or facility is used less than was anticipated, that is no proof that it is needed less than anticipated.

There is also the matter of the intensity of the physician's interaction. James and Herbert (1992) found that, even if certain interventions were more effective with specific patients, the more extensively the physician intervened, the higher was the probability that the patient would abstain, irrespective of their individual characteristics.

As the second variable let us consider concerns about the attitude and skills of the doctor. It seems to be a truism, and Ockene (1987) has shown it to be so, that the training of physicians has increased their effectiveness. Also

Fowler (1993) reports that training doctors in smoking cessation techniques can increase the likelihood of them advising patients to stop smoking, and thus increase their health promotion effectiveness. However, Richmond and Webster (1990) believe that most doctors lack the necessary training in smoking cessation counselling and this can lead to a 'self-fulfilling prophecy' in which doctors avoid health promotion activities and are pessimistic about smoking interventions.

The relative efficacy of nurses

Notwithstanding the wealth of research into doctors and smoking cessation programmes, there appears to be a dearth of such information relating to nurses. Government policy has recognised that nurses should play a major role in health promotion and the White Papers, *Promoting Better Health* (DHSS 1987) and *The Health of the Nation* (DOH 1992), in describing the role that all of the members of the primary health care team must occupy in health promotion, specify that nurses such as 'health visitors, community nurses and practice nurses' are 'well placed to promote good health and prevent ill health' (DHSS 1987). It is also acknowledged that the success of the key areas in 'the nation's health' will be dependent upon the 'commitment and skills' of 'nurses and health visitors' (DOH 1992). The clear assumption is that they already occupy a high profile in this context and that it should be enhanced.

Gott and O'Brian (1990) are of the view that policy-makers and educators have responded to these calls for nurses to be the leaders in health promotion, without first considering the legitimacy and development of this role in nursing. The indications are that nurses would seem to be enthusiastic about health promotion, and health visitors have always regarded themselves as health promoters first and foremost. But Gott (1990) argues that enthusiasm is not enough, because the leadership role in primary healthcare has always been assigned to doctors and not nurses, and that this is no different with health promotion.

As has already been shown, changes in healthcare policy have led to an increase in health promotion within primary healthcare, and yet Calnan and Williams (1993) have shown that the majority of this is carried out by practice nurses. One of the outcomes of their study was that the GP contract of 1990 has resulted directly in the employment of more nurses. In fact, the number of practice nurses in England and Wales has quadrupled since 1986 and there were 8,155 full-time equivalent practice nurses employed in 1990 (DOH 1990). The practice nurse is principally concerned with clinical work, which is analogous to the consultation mode of the GP (Calnan and Williams 1993). While the new contract, which heralds a shift from group and clinic work to a one-to-one approach, may increase the doctor's involvement, Stilwell (1991) nevertheless believes that the practice nurse has now an established and firm position within primary healthcare.

In this connection, a study by Sanders *et al.* (1989) dealt a devastating blow to practice nurses involved in health promotion. It showed that the effect of nurse intervention in smoking cessation was minimal! Moreover, this finding has been replicated in more recent studies by both OXCHECK (1994) and The Family Heart Study Group (1994). In each of these studies, general practitioners were supported by nurses trained to screen and intervene. The OXCHECK study was mounted two years before the original GP contract and entailed a four-year block randomised evaluation of the health checks offered by practice nurses. On the other hand, The British Family Heart Study Group was a randomised controlled trial in general practices in thirteen towns in Britain, whose aim was to measure the impact of the programmes of cardiovascular screening and lifestyle intervention led by nurses. Thus the studies were qualitatively different. However, the results of both studies have shown that the general health checks offered by nurses have been ineffective in helping smokers to stop smoking and there has been no significant change in smoking rates.

While these disappointing results need not necessarily be interpreted as a failure in the ability of the practice nurse to undertake health promotion, they may well reflect the way in which health promotion is both perceived and carried out within the primary health teams.

For example, a study by Bradford and Winn (1993) which surveyed the practice nurses' view of health promotion found that, although the GP contract emphasised the performance of health promotion duties, in reality much of the nurse's time was devoted to treatment-orientated activities. This study also highlighted the fact that 75 per cent of those practice nurses questioned felt that they needed more health promotion training.

All of this parallels the findings of Macleod Clark *et al.* (1985) which suggest that nurses' baseline knowledge levels are inadequate or inappropriate for undertaking the 'education' role in smoking advice and that, although nurses recognise their potential health education role, they lack the knowledge and skills to carry them out effectively. They also are aware of this deficiency and wish to overcome it. This, of course, has financial and personnel resource implications if it is going to be remedied. It also suggests a continuing role for one day a week part-time health promotion courses.

More recently a study by Ross *et al.* (1994) highlights the wide variety of work and increasing responsibility of practice nurses, who still practise within a climate of ill-defined roles and limited educational and training possibilities. Importantly this study also brought into sharp relief the 'mismatch between training and practice'.

Subsequently, further research, by Macleod Clark *et al.* in 1987, employed a case study approach to analyse sixty-eight nurse-initiated health education interventions related to smoking cessation. It indicated quite the reverse, namely, that nurse intervention may be just as effective as that of doctors and it reported, moreover, that 60 per cent of the sample were 'influenced' in some way by the nurse. The study design was unique in that it attempted to link the outcome of the intervention to the actual process. Additionally, it subsequently suggests that it is effective communication skills and client involvement that is central to success, rather than just advice and information giving.

A singular feature of this study, though, was the composition of the sample. Of the sixteen nurses involved, seven were health visitors, six were midwives and three were ward nurses, so that, although the majority of the nurses were involved in primary care, practice nurses were not included at all in the sample. In that respect, then, the characteristics and motivation of the patients involved in this intervention, and the environment in which the intervention was offered, contrast to the more usual smoking cessation activity carried out in the GP's surgery. Almost half (47 per cent) of Macleod Clark's sample were found to be worried about the effects of their smoking on their babies and all had previously agreed to discuss smoking with the nurse, thus indicating a significant motivation for the intervention. This compares unfavourably with the opportunistic approach of the health check, when the practice nurse, along with all of the other medical procedures, advises patients to stop smoking.

Macleod Clark et al. (1987) do cite training as being imperative to successful intervention and, as health visitors and midwives have additional training, perhaps it could be surmised that training in health promotion is the required prerequisite to effective health promotion activity. Indeed, this is borne out by the study by Ross et al. (1994), in whose sample of practice nurses only 19 per cent had a formal training in primary care nursing (health visiting or district nursing qualification). The conclusion was reached that the majority of practice nurses 'have only a limited knowledge base of epidemiology, public health, health promotion and nursing care in non-institutional settings' and that the majority of nurses in this sample wanted further training. The RCN (1984) and Stilwell (1991) have also acknowledged the problems associated with lack of organised training for practice nurses. This further strengthens the argument for funding part-time training for practice nurses in health promotion.

The role of psychology in smoking cessation programmes

The DOH publication, *Better Living, Better Life* (1993a), acknowledged that, in order to achieve effective intervention, health professionals should be aware of the important contribution of health psychology, because it enables practitioners to employ techniques 'more successful than the traditional approaches of advice-giving' (DOH 1993a) which will better motivate patients to change their behaviour.

The publication in question outlines a 'Practice Plan for Effective Interventions' for smoking cessation, that replicates the conditions described by Damrosch (1991) as being most likely to change health-related behaviour. Damrosch defends the view that change is most likely to occur when patients perceive that the threat to their health and to their own vulnerability is high; but that their ability to mediate the appropriate change in their behaviour and the effectiveness of that response is equally high. This 'double high/double efficacy' model is drawn from several psychology-based sources. The main three influences are the 'Health Belief Model' (HBM), Bandura's self-efficacy model and research concerning fear appeals. All, of course, rely on the conscious enhancement of self-esteem and autonomy and thus have a positive impact on empowerment.

It is not the author's remit here to evaluate these different approaches to change motivation, but it is important to briefly consider them as a justification for the range of strategies that may be employed within primary healthcare teams from smoking cessation programmes, beyond that of advice giving, and within a truly health promotion context.

The Health Belief Model, of course, is the most researched theory of intervention and DiNicola and DiMatteo (1984) believe that it can be used to predict an individual's intentions to practise health-related behaviours. Although it has been criticised for its failure to consider other factors that may affect motivation, one of these being the addictive nature of cigarette smoking (Janz and Becker 1984), it does highlight the need for health promoters to consider an individual's attitudes and beliefs in some detail before embarking on a specific smoking cessation programme.

From the foregoing, therefore, it is evident that empowerment is an important concept in smoking cessation, as it establishes the connection between knowledge and action; because the belief that one can carry out a preferred behaviour usually occurs before one actually attempts the behaviour. Bandura (1986) defined this empowerment as a 'self-efficacy – a judgement of one's capacity to accomplish a certain level of performance'. He posits that this kind of self-judgement is based on four information sources:

1   the individual's own performance;
2   the experience and performance of others;
3   the persuasiveness of the health promoter;
4   the psychological evidence the individual can gain from their own behaviour or performance.

This has immense implications for practice, and Bandura cited the importance of using evidence from all four sources of information to 'provide helpful guides for implementing programmes of personal change' (1986). Most critically, the relevance of this concept to practice resides in its ability to predict behaviour, which has the capacity to identify high-risk situations in which the individual may feel unable to cope, in order that an appropriate intervention may take place.

Exhortation used to constitute a much more dominant part of the old health education programmes. In the 1950s one could say that fear and behaviour change fuelled and undergirded methods of health education. Much of this was squarely based, no doubt, on the study by Janis and Feshbach (1953). Clearly, excessive use of fear is counterproductive, but it still has a role to play, provided that it is within a context which respects the person's autonomy. Although there does not seem to be any clear consistency in subsequent research about how this is done, Job (1988) has outlined how low-level fear, combined with short-term rewards and specific skill teaching, can be used in helping people to stop smoking, and he describes three ways in which fear can be used effectively to stop people smoking:

1   A low-level of fear should be used where emphasis is upon immediate physical effects, such as blood pressure reduction.
2   Short-term reinforcers should be used, such as increased efficiency in climbing stairs.
3   The health promoter should teach the individual skills required to aid the giving up process, in preference to only giving specific advice.

In practical terms, the findings of this attitude-change research are invaluable to practitioners, as their application to practice should ensure 'effective interventions designed to motivate health related behaviour change' (Damrosch 1991).

Also of great relevance is another model related to behaviour change, as described by Prochaska and DiClemente (1984). The 'Stages of Change' model is referred to in the Health Education Authority's training course for practice nurses and is considered to be most relevant to smoking behaviour. Initial failure is assumed and the model is based on the assumptions that, for many, success is only achieved after several attempts and that, by adopting a client-centred approach, the patient will receive an intervention appropriate to their stage of change. Brownell *et al.* (1986) offer detailed strategies for achieving maximum effectiveness and these strategies form a basis for the broad guide-lines offered by the *Better Living Better Life* document.

All of these findings emphatically underline the need for an individualised approach to change behaviour programmes, in which knowledge of health psychology assists the practitioner to more effectively carry out health promotion activity. This places it unequivocally in the realm of health promotion. Indeed, this would seem to be acknowledged by the NHS Management Executive who, in its 1993 document on the implementation of the GP contracts, advises GPs to use a practice plan or protocol in the implementation of smoking cessation programmes. Going on to confirm the need for and the requirement of practitioners to be fully informed of relevant research findings, this document demonstrates evidence of their application in practice in order that their health promotion activity achieves maximum effectiveness.

13

USE AND ABUSE OF ALCOHOL: A HEALTH PROMOTION PERSPECTIVE

Identifying the problem

Before its effectiveness can be evaluated, health promotion must be focused on to a problem. But the problem must be real and empirically defined. Consider alcohol abuse, it is recognised world-wide as a problem, and an immensely contrived series of legislative initiatives attempt to constrict it from every side, ranging from when one is allowed to sell alcohol, to sanctions against driving a vehicle with more than a certain alcohol level in the bloodstream. Even the WHO made alcohol abuse the subject of one of its thirty-eight targets for *Health for All* 2000 (1985), as follows:

> By 1995, in all Member States, there should be significant decrease in such health damaging behaviour as overuse of alcohol . . . . The attainment of this target could be significantly supported by developing integrated programmes aimed at reducing consumption of alcohol, and of other harmful substances, by at least 25% by the year 2000.

Nothing could appear more straightforward. However, in this chapter the author will demonstrate some of the difficulties which would render health promotion initiatives in this area (an area which is perceived to be of immense importance) problematic.

Most of the difficulties stem from three sources:

1   the medical status of alcohol abuse;
2   selective use of models of alcohol use and abuse;
3   lack of coherent definitions.

Alcohol use and abuse are almost as old as civilisation itself but the matter has been, if anything, rendered more obscure on that account. The fact that some alcohol induced behaviour states come across as having an almost mystical and incantational quality probably has, over the years, encouraged irrational ways of looking at it. Indeed, today some people treat the biomedically explainable behaviour state induced by some drugs as having some sort of spiritual dimension.

Despite the vagary surrounding explicit definitions of alcohol abuse and of alcoholism, however, their impact on society is very real and accurately measurable. The social cost, which includes the strictly financial cost, is altogether enormous and it is very much a legitimate concern for the health promotion worker. But the lack of unambiguous definition – when does heavy or frequent drinking become alcohol abuse and when does alcohol abuse become alcoholism? – renders empowerment an entirely different proposition.

Trying to isolate an unambiguous context

The tempting idea that there is a single cause for alcohol-related problems, or even an easily identifiable cluster of causes, has no support in the literature (Velleman 1992). As shall be discussed later, risk factors can be statistically isolated. A dominant approach today, and certainly one that is widely accepted as being legitimate among lay people, is the idea of alcohol misuse as being a 'disease'. Such a view has many merits. It removes the heavy onus of 'victim blaming'. It encourages compassion and discourages opprobrium. It highlights a national search for solutions rather than punishment of the victim. Finally, it confers a high profile on neighbourhood support for the victim's family. With all of that going for it, it is a shame that the 'disease model' has not attracted more empirical support. The problem remains that, in most human societies, almost every adult drinks alcohol and in amounts in excess of quantities which have proven the downfall of a few. How frustratingly unlike cigarette smoking this all is.

Velleman (1992), in his sound account of counselling about alcohol intake problems, is driven to the definition: 'Problematic drinking is drinking that causes problems!' If, in desperate search for something more empirical, we look to the *Diagnostic and Statistical Manual II* (revised) (*DSM II R*), manual of the American Psychiatric Association (1988), we find abuse of alcohol divided into three categories, as follows:

1 the regular daily consumption of 'large amounts' of alcohol;
2 regular drinking bouts, with no drinking between them, such as 'weekend binges';
3 irregular and seemingly unpredictable periods of heavy drinking lasting several days or weeks, interspersed with weeks or months of normal, predictable and sober behaviour.

Later in this chapter we shall consider Hutcheson's (1988) criteria applied to alcohol use in the British context, but from a different perspective.

Lacking in empirical rigour as these categories are, they come across as starkly reductionist in the context of the *DSM II R*'s further elaborations on them. They claim that: 'It is a mistake to regard these patterns as in any sense definitive or to associate any one of them exclusively with a condition designated as "alcoholism"'. They do isolate one 'species' of alcoholism, known as 'gamma alcoholism', as being associated principally with a loss of control. The victim drinks with no intellectual or cognitive control over the amount ingested. This 'gamma alcoholism' is the stereotype most lay people have in mind when they think of the 'alcoholic'. In fact, the well-known support group, Alcoholics Anonymous, was started in the US and its methods directed exclusively at that type of alcoholism. However, there are other types.

Biomedical literature generally has tried to reflect an analytical approach to the problem by reporting investigations on such phenomena as alcohol tolerance, dependence and withdrawal syndromes. The latter have proven to be especially useful, the severity of the withdrawal syndrome being held to be an index of the strength of the original 'alcoholism'.

Ascertaining levels of alcohol addiction

The viewpoint of the National Institute of Alcohol Abuse and Alcoholism of the USA is that there are some specific mechanisms – phenomena that are indicative of addiction to alcohol.

First of all there is reinforcement, either positive or negative. Positive reinforcement is about the repetition of an action (in our case of drinking alcohol) because it brings pleasure or some other kind of reward and it is theorised that this process established the drug (alcohol) seeking behaviour. After that establishment, and with the passing of time, the human brain succeeds in functioning adequately under the presence of alcohol, but then it cannot adapt immediately to the withdrawal of alcohol. That lack leads to the withdrawal symptoms, indicative of the already established dependence. In physiological terms, a threshold blood alcohol level is gradually established below which some of the normal physiological processes, including many associated with such automatic processes as homoeostasic maintenance, cannot be carried out. What is suggested in this model is that 'addiction' actually implies an alteration of the biomedical/physiological signals which mediate the processes concerned. While such interpretations may explain why that should happen to some people's biochemistry but not to that of most of us, 'sickness' or 'disease' is not a particularly good taxonomic for it – the aetiology is too general and not exclusive and, while risk behaviours can be isolated, causes defy analysis. What we do know, though, is that once addiction is established, the attempt to withdraw from it can best be described in behavioural terms as 'negative reinforcement' (*Alcohol Alert 33* 1996). Therefore, drinking becomes 'necessary' to avoid the pain of withdrawal. This motivation to avoid that painful stage is the negative reinforcement (*Alcohol Alert 33* 1996).

Drummond (1991) in his study about dependence refers to some similar elements about the dependence syndrome in general, such as increased tolerance to the drug, repeated withdrawal symptoms, subjective awareness of compulsion to take the drug, salience of drug-seeking behaviour, relief or avoidance of withdrawal symptoms, narrowing of the repertoire of drug taking, and reinstatement following a period of abstinence.

West (1991), examining the psychological theories of addiction, suggests that there are three main theoretical orientations:

1   the aversive consequences of abstinence (withdrawal avoidance theories);
2   the positive attributes of the behaviour (appetitive theories);
3   distortion of the motivational process itself (motivational distortion theories).

Alternative models

There are a number of objections to this type of paradigm. For instance, the literature is replete with accounts of people who, having been detoxicated successfully for many years, suddenly re-experience the craving, even though the biomedical contextual basis for the sort of physiological dependence described previously should by then have reversed. This would seem to suggest that there is some other factor (or factors) involved and an explanation available which transcends the narrowly biochemical.

To avoid a high level of reductionism, other models have been proposed. Consider the 'appetitive' model. This focuses on the positive effects of the drug, suggesting that it is its pleasant affect which creates the conditions for subsequent dependency and addiction. In that view, alcohol helps the user to cope with stress, and the most obvious aspect of not reacting to what might, in reasonable terms, be regarded as a 'stressful' situation, is a behaviour reflecting less concern with the future and a higher level of impulsive action.

Then, again, there are various motivational disorder models that consider addiction in even more psychological, rather than physiological, terms as a dimension of 'habit strength'. In those interpretations, 'habit strength' refers to the causal association between a stimulus, which is a cue to an action, and the subsequent action itself. However, these models are not a great deal of help in objectifying the discourse, because the mechanism by which repetition of an action in the presence of the stimulus then strengthens this link is not made clear.

West (1991) lastly concludes that each one of these theories accounts for some features of addiction. It has been proposed that in most of the cases there is an involvement of more than one mechanism. A model that explains addiction more broadly in all of its range has still to be enunciated.

The biggest question that arises is: What causes alcohol-related problems? What is to blame for problem drinking?

Ascertaining causes

In general there are two hugely embrasive categories of causes related to alcohol abuse; causes that refer to the individual (factors within the individual) and causes that refer to the social environment of the individual (factors within the social context). The first tend to focus on the physiological/biochemical while the latter tend to draw heavily on the psychological. As Velleman (1992) states, the first category is based on the belief that the reason why some people develop problems with their drinking has something to do with them as individuals. The idea that the problem drinker has 'got something' which 'normal' people do not has been around for a long time (Velleman 1992). But to that category could be assigned a non-behaviourist cluster, namely the old theory about allergy to alcohol, and these aim, with the more psychological models, the psychiatric illness conception, the alcoholic personality theory and even theories about genetic predisposition, to provide a rational basis for responding to the issue.

The allergy to alcohol theory suggests that people with problem drinking suffer from an allergy that does not let them control their drinking, so that they evidence a craving to drink continuously and incontrollably. However, there is not one shred of evidence to back it up (Velleman 1992). It is paradoxical, therefore, that such a model, which seems primitive in comparison with more recent theories, has affected to such a great degree the current dominant beliefs that alcoholism is a disease.

That mainly happened due to the adaptation of that theory by the co-founder of the American Alcoholics Anonymous, Bill Willson. Willson was influenced by Dr William Silkworth (who was a client). Silkworth, after the First World War, was one of the first to treat alcoholics as though they were allergic to alcohol. Because of the historical–social conditions (Prohibition was repealed in the US in 1933) the AA (Alcoholics Anonymous), that had begun in 1935, grew rapidly. The initial Silkworth/Willson model was transmitted through the AA communities and with the passing of time became the dominant US conception of alcoholism, namely, that of a progressive incurable disease, which is accepted by 90 per cent of Americans (Peele 1993; Wells 1991).

Treating alcohol problems as mental illness

The psychiatric illness approach is based on the idea that alcoholism is a mental disorder and that it should be treated according to the symptomology and the history of the patient (Velleman 1992; Belle-Glass and Marshall 1991).

The alcoholic personality approach itself has two versions. This first is based on the assumption that if a person abuses alcohol for many years, his or her personality alters and he or she then acquires a new alcoholic personality. The second version suggests that there is a type of personality that is itself a great predispositional factor for some people to develop problems with alcohol (Velleman 1992).

Finally a number of studies have been published about the genetic predisposition that some people have to either develop alcoholism as such, or to acquire problems related to alcohol. This would give credence to the idea that all offspring of alcoholic parents have a greater possibility of becoming alcoholic themselves. Such statistical indications have led many to the conclusion that there is such a genetic contribution to alcoholism. We can refer, for instance, to research in Scandinavia during the 1960s and 1970s (e.g. Kaji 1966; Partanen *et al.* 1966). These first studies focused on the comparison of concordance rates of alcoholism among monozygotic versus dizygotic twins. Prevalence of alcohol problems among separated monozygotic twins would indicate that there is a genetic predisposition for such problems.

Other studies focused on half-siblings and adoptees. Schuckit (1987) found that 20 per cent of the half-siblings of hospitalised alcoholics were also alcoholics. Cadoret and Gath (1978) found that, even if a son of alcoholic parents has been raised by non-alcoholics (adoptive) parents, that does not reduce his greater probability of becoming an alcoholic himself.

Even if these theories are proven true, it still only addresses a small part of the complex question of alcohol abuse and of alcoholism. Aspects such as the lifestyle and the environment (social and cultural) may well be the only factors that determine who is going to be a problematic drinker and who is not.

Social and environmental influences with respect to problem drinking have already been epidemiologically established as 'risk-factors', of course. It is in this context that personal insight (attendant upon self-esteem) and psycho-social awareness can be pivotal in the successful resolution of such problems, and these are also the attributes definitive of empowerment in health promotion.

Paramount among these influences is the family. Clearly the family plays a very important role in the socialisation of people and its function or dysfunction affects all its members, especially the juveniles. For that reason a dysfunctional family has long been considered as the number one risk factor in the development of problematic drinking, especially for the children and adolescents. There is ample statistical support for the view that children need extra care because the links between childhood encounters with these problems (especially when they are unresolved) establish the necessary clinical preconditions for adult alcohol abuse (Oyemade and Washington 1990). Obviously critical in this regard are family values and child-rearing practices. Families that employ negative and authoritarian discipline, with no stable rules other than the arbitrary parental will, experience more problems in preventing adolescent alcohol abuse. On the contrary, families which operate under stable and positive rules are less likely to have children who are alcohol abusers (Oyemade 1985). Other important risk factors related to the family, naturally enough, centre on such factors as one-parent families, frequent family disagreements, poor communications and unclear expectations of parents (Delgado 1990). One of the most influential family risk factors is the alcoholism/alcohol abuse of parents or siblings (Zeitlin and Swadi 1991).

Again, the influence of peer groups has been established as crucial (Zeitlin and Swadi 1991). O'Connor (1978) suggests that peer group pressure mainly determines the incorporation of alcohol consumption into lifestyles of adolescents. Generally, and not only for the adolescents, there is the well-known tendency of compliance with the attitudes of the group. For example, Peele (1996) suggests that drinking in male-dominated bars is considerably heavier than drinking during meals with one's family.

Lack of social competence has been identified as a causal factor in the abuse of alcohol. If the social environment is excessively competitive and stressful, leading an individual to repeated coping failure, alcohol abuse is a common enough response. This happens because alcohol may appear as itself a safe and sociably acceptable way to cope with stress (Freeman 1990). The WHO (1986) has argued that the key here is to block the transformation of such temporary alcohol abuse from assuming the status of a lifestyle pattern.

Poverty and low socio-economic status have also been established as being risk factors. Poverty affects both directly and indirectly the abuse of alcohol; directly because it is connected with low self-esteem and self-respect and indirectly because of its consequences to family and its connection with underclass. Labouvie (1986) found that a growing sense of powerless or helplessness is a prominent indicative factor for alcohol abuse by adolescents and Nobles et al. (1987) suggest that poor self-esteem is a key risk factor for substance abuse.

There are also a wide variety of psychodynamic factors, arising from the interaction between the social context and the individual, that have been regarded as causative of frequent substance abuse. Among there are: rebelliousness (Kandel 1982), non-conformity to traditional values (Jessor and Jessor 1977), high tolerance of deviance, resistance to authority, strong need for independence and normlessness (Jessor and Jessor 1975).

In all these, the potential for health promotion to play a positive role is obviously enormous. Let us now consider and analyse actual community health promotion initiatives directed at such problems in Britain.

Health promotion as an agency in addressing the problem

It is evident that the notion of partnership, public participation, and collaboration are seen to be integral to health promotion. These factors are all important to any concept of a multi-agency strategy for the reduction of alcohol misuse. A broad health promotion plan towards the prevention of alcohol misuse must assume a holistic approach. It would need to consider all of these factors and, in addition, would have to include education, legal, fiscal/economic and environmental measures which are all part of the process of 'building healthy public policy'.

Within health promotion there are a number of models employed which have already been considered. Thus, Tones (1990) regards health promotion as a 'preventive model', the goal being to persuade the individual to assume more responsible decisions, i.e. to adopt behaviours which will prevent disease. The concern is to produce behavioural outcomes, and health education will only have been effective if individuals or communities demonstrate that they have adopted a more healthy lifestyle. Examples of the prevention of alcohol misuse using this model may include media campaigns to reinforce attitudes and behaviour change, better labelling of alcohol content in drinks, the Health Education Authorities' 'Drinkwise Campaign' and leaflets and other information which increase knowledge of the harmful effects of alcohol misuse.

This model has, however, been criticised as it ignores the real socio-political roots of ill-health and can lead to victim blaming. Crawford 1977 (cited in Tones 1990) argues, for example, that it is inefficient and unethical to blame the victim for adopting an unhealthy lifestyle when society itself creates an environment which sustains the unhealthy habits health education seeks to eliminate.

Secondly, Tones (1990) discusses the radical-political model, the goal of this model being to get to the roots of the problem of alcohol abuse. This model is concerned to achieve social and environmental change by triggering political action. Examples of action toward the prevention of alcohol misuse may include activities such as campaigns for changes in licensing laws and calls for increases in the real price of alcohol. Tones (1990) specifies that the evaluation of this model would mean health educators would have to demonstrate, at the least, a heightened level of awareness or of critical consciousness. Ideally a consciousness-raising programme would also lead to measurable action.

The third model of health promotion as described by Tones (1990) is the self-empowerment model. In its simplest form, this model would consist merely of providing knowledge, success therefore being relatively easy to define and to achieve. This model rests on the assumption that knowledge is sufficient to facilitate informed decision-making. Examples of good practice in health promotion activity would therefore include the distribution of leaflets such as 'Cut Down on your Drinking' and 'Drink Wisely'. It is known, however, that knowledge alone is insufficient and because of this a more sophisticated version of the model argues that knowledge should be supplemented by non-traditional teaching methods which would ensure the clarification of values underlying decision-making and would also provide an opportunity to practise decision-making. Self-help groups, such as Alcoholics Anonymous, could therefore be considered in this context.

As illustrated, any of these approaches might be employed to address alcohol consumption and alcohol misuse. Bennett (1994) claims professional and ideological preferences may determine the approach used but that often a variety of different types of interventions are employed in respect of alcohol misuse.

The British context and its implications for health promotion

The problem of alcohol misuse is often referred to as one of the greatest public health problems of Britain, yet as a nation we have been slow to recognise the growing threat that alcohol poses to health, partly because alcohol is such an integral part of British culture. According to the Health Education Authority (HEA) (1993) in *Health Update 3: Alcohol*, over 90 per cent of Britains drink and most do so without apparently damaging themselves or others.

Problem drinking used to be seen as a practice confined to a small minority of the population who were known as 'alcoholics'. However, in *The Nation's Health*, Hutcheson (1988) argues that this is now known not to be the case as there are three identifiable kinds of problem drinking, of which alcohol dependence forms only a small proportion. The Office of Health Economics 1981 (cited in Hutcheson 1988) lists the three categories as being:

1 Heavy drinking (showing biochemical abnormality) – 3 million are estimated to be at risk.
2 Problem drinking (causes harm to the drinker and others) – approximately 700,000.
3 Alcohol dependence – approximately 150,000.

While research confirms that the heaviest drinkers are individually at most risk of harm, Kreitman (1986, cited in Hutcheson 1988) suggests that the biggest burden of alcohol-related ill-health is to be found among those who are less heavy drinkers, as they are more numerous. From this it can be suggested that health promotion in terms of the prevention of alcohol misuse should be targeted towards the community as a whole, rather than focusing on a small, high-risk minority which is likely to be difficult to reach.

Tones (1987) argues that, when attempting to decrease alcohol misuse, it is important to understand the various psycho-social and environmental factors which contribute to health-related decision-making. A number of models employed in health promotion attempt to explain how people make health related decisions, but Tones' 'Health Action Model' provides an overview of these influences and could be extremely useful for developing relevant health promotion strategies directed at alcohol abuse.

Extent of the problem

In Britain Saunders (1984) states that over the past 300 years marked fluctuations in consumption of alcohol have occurred, with periods of heavy use characterised by cheap and easily available alcohol and high rates of drunkenness and morbidity.

The Royal College of Psychiatrists (1986) in *Alcohol Our Favourite Drug* trace patterns of consumption in Britain and illustrate how, after 1900, consumption of alcohol began to fall due to various restrictions in opening times of licensed premises and controls on production. The end of the First World War was marked by a rise in consumption again, but it fell during the economic depression of the 1930s and remained comparatively low until the late 1950s. The fall in alcohol consumption, which began during the First World War, gave rise to the most sober period in British history and the three decades 1920–1950 clearly reflect the advantage of a diminishing per capita consumption. Taylor (cited in Saunders 1984) demonstrates statistically how the number of alcohol-related problems declined dramatically, with offences for drunkenness falling from 60/10,000 population (1912) to 10/10,000 population in 1932. Mortality figures were affected and deaths from alcoholism and liver cirrhosis fell, from approximately 150/million population (1912) to 35/million population (1932).

However, over the next quarter century, alcohol consumption practically doubled. The Health Education Authority (1993) illustrates how in Britain per capita alcohol consumption rose steeply in the 1970s followed by a decline between 1979 and 1983. Again, in 1991 the population drank 9.05 litres per capita. Such an increase in alcohol consumption over the past thirty years suggests that Britons, particularly the young, are increasingly valuing the use of alcohol as part of their leisure and recreational activities. Thomas *et al.* (1992), quoted in the 1992 *General Household Survey,* indicate that consumption is now highest by women and men in the younger age group.

It is not difficult to defend the view that a major cause of this trend must be that alcoholic beverages are being produced in continuously increasing quantities and are becoming more widely and readily available (Grant and Ritson 1983). The twenty years between 1960 and 1980 saw increases in production of 40 per cent for wine and 124 per cent for beer. Such alcoholic beverages are all relatively easy to produce, hence the constraints on production must lie principally in terms of what the market will consume. But that is also controlled by affordability, and alcohol in Britain is cheaper today in terms of available disposable income than it has ever been before.

As already observed, Saunders (1987) claims that one of the crucial factors which arises from studying British drinking history is that, as per capita consumption has risen and fallen, the indices of alcohol-related harm have done likewise. Thus, since we know that there has been a near doubling of alcohol use in the last thirty years, it is crucial that we try to limit alcohol consumption.

Empirical considerations

The Health Education Authority (1993) estimate that around 7 million adults are drinking at levels above the suggested 'sensible limits'. Sensible weekly limits were defined as up to twenty-one units of alcohol a week for men and up to fourteen units for women and were agreed by the Royal College of Psychiatrists, various other medical colleges, the HEA, Alcohol Concern and others, in what the *Sunday Observer* headlined as 'Medical Royal Colleges Consensus Calls for Increase in the Price of Alcohol' (19 November 1987: 2). Of course, these figures were modified slightly upward in 1996. One unit of alcohol is equivalent to one glass of wine or half a pint of ordinary strength beer.

Interestingly, a 1993 report suggests that alcohol consumption may actually now be decreasing. In a report entitled 'Britain's Flight from Alcohol', Williams (1993) examined trends in alcohol consumption 1985–1992 and stated that the situation in 1987 showed an increase in people who had chosen to abstain completely from alcohol. The remaining drinkers, however, seem to be consuming more alcohol than previously.

Williams (1993) claims that since 1987 the trend away from alcohol has increased and today 17.9 per cent of adults in the UK do not use alcohol, an increase of one-fifth on the 14 per cent figure recorded in 1985, which was used as a baseline for the study. Since he makes no reference as to whether the remaining drinkers are still drinking more than before or whether this too has decreased, this study can be said to be inconclusive. This is in contrast to other evidence, such as that from the 1995 *General Household Survey*, which showed that, over the last nine years, there has been very little change in the percentages of non-drinkers and moderate drinkers, although there has been an increase in the percentages drinking over the recommended levels of fourteen and twenty-one units per week.

Strategies for reducing consumption

As already indicated, it is almost unanimously accepted that there is a fixed relationship between the mean consumption of alcohol in a population and the prevalence of drinkers at certain levels of consumption. Ledermann first developed this view in 1956 (cited in Garretsen and Goor 1992) and it is now known as the 'single distribution model of alcohol use in a population'. The model strongly supports the idea that a reduction in the mean consumption level will result in a disproportionately large reduction in the category of heavy drinkers. In Britain, all three medical colleges and the WHO, among many, have accepted the evidence that the amount of damage from alcohol in a community correlated closely with the total amount consumed by that community.

However, there is disagreement as to how levels of consumption should be decreased in order to limit the amount of alcohol-related harm. Some have argued that this is not a task for health educators at all, but for politicians. For example, Dillner (1991) states that, given the evidence above, the most effective way to reduce the harm associated with alcohol must be to raise the price so as, in effect, to reduce the availability of alcohol and she argues that it is a job for politicians. The Lothian study by Kendell *et al.* (1983) has indeed lent support to the idea that an increase in price will result in a reduction of consumption for heavy drinkers as much as for light drinkers.

As well, the WHO (1985) in *Targets for Health for All* have historically recognised the importance of price policies and of other factors, such as regulations concerning production and advertisement policies. To ascertain precisely the relationship between advertising and alcohol consumption level, research has been done. But studies such as those by Ogborne and Smart (1980) have found that restrictions of advertising have been neither fully credible nor effective. Again, more controlled studies of restricted advertising, such as Wilcox (1985 cited in Bennett and Anthony 1992), have also proved ineffective. After critically analysing the evidence on advertising and alcohol consumption, Duffy (1981 cited in Bennett and Anthony 1992) has concluded that the real price of alcohol does remain a much more powerful deterrent.

Despite this, it is argued by several writers that major price adjustment is extremely unlikely to happen, whatever party is in government. An obvious reason for this is that, although alcohol misuse costs society a great deal, there are also many benefits to alcohol use. In Britain, for example, the production, marketing and selling of alcoholic beverages employs in excess of three-quarters of a million people (Saunders 1992). As well, the alcohol production industry is efficient, profitable and a substantial investor in plant and machinery, with exports of alcohol exceeding £1,000 million per annum. He argues that it is hardly surprising, therefore, that governments have taken no significant steps to decrease alcohol consumption and it would be even more surprising if they did decide to in the future.

Such fiscal considerations are also emphasised by Dillner (1991), who claims that it is also true that at least fifteen government departments are thought to have alcohol interests, many of which are concerned with increasing consumption rather than with limiting it. Since the drinks industry is a very powerful ally of the government, it is therefore unlikely that the latter will implement regulations to restrict their output. In that case, therefore, action must come from other sources, but still not necessarily health educators, according to some authors. What is really needed is an energetic political campaign with an organisation like ASH at its centre which has been so successful in reducing levels of smoking (Dillner 1991).

How might health promoters see the problem?

For instance, many would argue that action at a national level, to the exclusion of anything else, is misguided, for the implication is that any response is the responsibility of central government. To accept such an argument would be to tacitly imply that health promotion does not have a great part to play in reducing alcohol consumption levels.

A possible reason for such a negative line of thought may be that, in the past, alcohol education has often been considered to be ineffective. But in the past, argues Roberts (1988), health education campaigns often concentrated on providing information alone. We now know that such an approach is almost certainly ineffective.

Additionally the literature is ambiguous on the matter and many lay people are confused. For example, while being told about the importance of monitoring our alcohol intake, reports are simultaneously published stating that alcohol may actually help to prevent heart disease.

According to Roberts (1988), another cause of ineffectiveness in alcohol education is that it has often been concentrated at the micro level and is thus frequently isolated from the full context of the problem. Alcohol education, he argues, is too preoccupied with focusing on enabling individuals to make informed choices. But it is his view that far more productive measures would be for health educators to concentrate their efforts on achieving the implementation of community measures, such as a complete ban on alcohol advertising, fiscal policies to keep high the real price of alcohol and measures such as the criminalisation of drunken driving, and random breath testing. In this, of course, he is advocating health promotion. The extent to which these measures would be successful, however, have not been well researched.

Assessing the effectiveness of interventions

Cohort analyses in alcohol misuse have been undertaken to ascertain whether alcohol education is effective and, in general, they have shown favourable results. One example is the York District Hospital (YDH) study by Rowland *et al.* (1992, cited in Rowland and Maynard 1993) in which early interventions did not appear to have any impact on drinking habits.

In this study, patients entering hospital identified as having been drinking to excess were divided into a control and intervention group, the intervention group being given an alcohol education pack consisting of a tape-slide presentation and an HEA booklet. A year later, although some of the patients who had received the alcohol education had fewer alcohol-related health problems, there were no further differences. In this case, therefore, standardised alcohol education did not affect consumption or improve knowledge about alcohol. There are several reasons why this could be, for example the nature of the intervention itself, the fact that it was carried out on a less personal basis than some of the other early intervention studies, or the patients may not have been concerned enough about their health, believing perhaps that their drinking was not at harmful levels. Such a finding sharply differentiates health education and health promotion and suggests the need for the latter.

As well, other studies, such as those by Skinner and Holt 1983 (cited in Rowland and Maynard 1993; Babor and Willetts 1986; and Chick *et al.* 1985), have shown that a minimal intervention to control drinking can be effective. Two examples given by Babor and Willetts (1986) are the Malmo Project in Sweden by Kristenson *et al.* 1982, 1983 (cited in Babor and Willetts 1986) and the Edinburgh Royal Infirmary Project, Scotland (cited in Babor and Willetts 1986). These projects both split patients with a raised level of serum glutamyltransferase (SGT) (which is an indication of alcohol abuse) into a control group and an intervention group. In the Swedish project, the intervention group were offered appointments with a physician every three months and a nurse every month until the SGT levels were normal. In the Edinburgh project those in the intervention group were given a 30–60 minute counselling session and a booklet giving advice on reducing drinking. Follow-up studies in both projects showed that the brief intervention led to a positive effect on drinking habits and physical health. These studies may have been more successful due to the longer duration of the intervention and the more personal basis on which the sessions were carried out. That is, they both gave expression to factors associated with inculcating a sense of personal worth (self-esteem) and dignity, and thus linked their outcomes to empowerment.

'Drinkwise' as a health promotion strategy

The HEA has set out to reduce the problem of alcohol misuse by the promotion of the 'sensible drinking' message which aims to encourage people to drink within the recommended weekly limits. Drinkwise campaigns, which take place on an annual basis, do claim to have had some impact on increasing awareness of the message and of the risks associated with alcohol use. The 'Beliefs About Alcohol' survey 1989 which was not published (cited in Alcohol Concern 1991) showed that just under half of the population had heard of the terms 'sensible drinking' and 'units of alcohol' (47 per cent and 46 per cent). The first two Drinkwise campaigns had raised these levels to 67 per cent (units) and 51 per cent (sensible limits). The proportion correctly identifying sensible weekly limits rose in 1990 from 6 per cent (men and women) to 10 per cent (men) and 8 per cent (women). The HEA 1992 Drinkwise campaign evaluation (cited in Health Education Authority 1993) among adults aged 16–54 found that 90 per cent claimed to be aware of the term 'units of alcohol'. Smaller percentages were able to display knowledge of the correct number of units in drinks measures.

However, while people may be aware of the levels of sensible drinking, they do not necessarily apply these levels to their own drinking. Additionally, any research which aims to establish personal drinking levels is subject to a relatively high degree of under reporting.

The effectiveness of general alcohol education campaigns is extremely difficult to ascertain. It is maintained by Alcohol Concern (1991) that there is still an unacceptably high level of complacency about drinking problems. Their research shows that nearly two-thirds of the population (64 per cent) think alcohol dangerous only if people become dependent on it. There is a high awareness of the increased health risks at certain specific levels of consumption, but awareness of specific values of the units and limits remains low. Also the claim that the HEA's 'Beliefs About Alcohol' survey (cited in Alcohol Concern 1991) shows similar results.

All of this would indicate that there is a place for health promotion in the prevention of alcohol misuse. It is especially evident that one of the most promising approaches which has emerged from studies of the data is that of community-based interventions, such as the Stanford Project 1972 and the North Karelia Project 1972 (cited in Bennett and Hodgson 1992).

Impact of the community

Neighbourhood advocacy and the importance of the community has received increasing attention in health promotion due in part to the growing recognition that behaviour is greatly influenced by the environment in which people live. As the Ottawa Charter 1986 states (cited in Green and Raeburn 1990):

Health promotion works through concrete and effective community action in setting priorities, making decisions, planning strategies and implementing them to achieve better health. At the heart of this process is the empowerment of communities, their ownership and control of their own endeavours and destinies.

Community-based projects demonstrated the potential effectiveness of multifaceted, integrated strategies and how behaviour change is more likely to occur when a variety of strategies are employed. For example, both the Stanford and North Karelia projects (cited in Bennett and Hodgson 1992) focus on modifying the major lifestyle risk factors leading to coronary heart disease. In the North Karelia project, there was an emphasis on community participation and attempts to change the environment. Its stated aim was to reduce levels of smoking, as assessed by lowering the serum cholesterol concentration and raised blood pressure values among the population. At the level of interface with the public, the programme included giving information to the people, integrating the programme into existing services and creating

174

any necessary new services, training health personnel and collecting data. When results were analysed, it was found, among other things, that over the period studied, the decrease in risk factors was generally greater than in the control community. It was the community-based approach, and integration of the activities, which were believed to have contributed most to the success of the project.

Therefore, both of these projects have provided convincing evidence to suggest that community-based approaches to health promotion can be effective in modifying health behaviour, especially if citizens are actively involved. Indeed, the WHO, on the basis of this evidence, recommended that it might be useful to deal with alcohol in the context of an overall health promotion approach throughout the community.

Public health through health promotion

In recent years, this type of approach has been referred to in the literature as 'multi-agency' working or 'healthy alliances' and it has received much publicity. Many perceive it as being a key solution to a host of public health problems. Hope for financial and resource support from the government for this type of working in terms of the prevention of alcohol misuse was given credence by the DOH (1989) in the Health Circular HN (89) 4 *Alcohol Misuse*, in which the Government stated that it was concerned about the effects of alcohol misuse. It then gave advice about the ways in which local organisations, with the support of the Government, could work together to combat the problem. In the *Health Circular* it was stated that: 'policy co-ordination nationally needs to be matched with local co-operation, with local organisations working together to: (i) identify local needs and (ii) decide how these can best be met'.

The DOH goes on to make suggestions about the way organisations might work together and gives examples of good practice which might be adopted.

None other than the Government's own *Health of the Nation* from the DOH (1992) places a great deal of emphasis on the prevention of alcohol problems. The stated aim is to reduce the proportion of men drinking more than 21 units of alcohol per week from 28 per cent in 1990 to 18 per cent by 2005 and the proportion of women drinking more than 14 units of alcohol per week from 11 per cent to 7 per cent. This section of the paper continues with a list of suggestions for reducing excessive alcohol ingestion, and then goes on to say: 'DHAs should seek to ensure that they are party to an agreed inter-agency alcohol misuse strategy'.

The Health Education Authority (1991) also gives support for local alcohol strategies in its response to the *Health of the Nation*, the WHO's Regional Office for Europe 1993 (cited in Rutherford 1993) and the Faculty of Public Medicine of the Royal College of Physicians (1991). It states as one of its targets to reduce alcohol related harm: 'By 2000 all health authorities and boards should develop a multi-agency community alcohol strategy . . . .'

A 'district or regional strategy' is a notion which draws support from the idea that, if a single multi-agency approach can be implemented, then services and resources can be more efficiently and effectively utilised to assess and meet local needs. Grant and Hodgson (1991), in *Responding to Drug and Alcohol Problems in the Community,* suggest ways in which a drug and alcohol strategy might be developed and implemented and argue that: 'active liaison between groups or organisations must be encouraged if the recent world-wide escalation in the problem of alcohol and drug abuse is to be reversed'.

Bennett and Anthony (1992) emphasise the above argument, stating that raising the alcohol awareness and promoting sensible drinking is an essential health promotion activity. Indeed, because it is a health promotional undertaking, there is no reason why this activity should be restricted to the health services. It would be much more effectively mediated in the context of neighbourhood advocacy and local action. They acknowledge that good practice in the evaluation of this type of action is very scarce, but claim that experience suggests that the more agencies that are involved, the more pervasive and resourceful the campaigns will be. It is widely assumed that any alcohol intervention taken by one agency inevitably impacts upon another so that, consequently, agencies have a collective responsibility.

Recently Wallace (1993) carried out research on the subject. It was his aim to ascertain (by questionnaire) the number of regions and districts in the UK which had implemented an alcohol strategy and the number intending to do so. In that study, 27 per cent of districts reported having a strategy, 65 per cent did not, 2 per cent were unsure and 7 per cent did not reply. The most disadvantaged in this aspect, with no districts reporting having a strategy, was the south-east Thames region. With respect to the actual quality of those strategies which have been implemented, research so far is incomplete.

In the view of Wallace (1993), the advantages of multi-agency working is the enablement of people to meet and exchange ideas, common ownership, the prevention of duplication of effort and clarification of those taking responsibility. He suggests what he terms 'quality measures', i.e. factors which are likely to influence a multi-agency commitment to an alcohol strategy. Among these factors are: joint ownership, clearly agreed outcome measures and success criteria, wide consultation, and an agreement about availability of resources. The author of this paper believes that one measure of quality is that strategies should be developed by a multi-agency group and that the degree of commitment may be judged by the number of agencies involved. Other criteria, he suggests, should include the presence of an action plan and recommendations, the implementation of the strategy and an appointed group to oversee this. Once a district has implemented a strategy, the action plan needs to be monitored to ensure that recommendations are being carried out.

Defining the role of health promotion in addressing alcohol misuse

In attempting to reduce the extent of alcohol misuse, it is desirable to have some understanding of the factors involved and to have a theoretical framework which can act as a basis for practice. As we know, Tones (1990) stated that such a framework should explain how individuals make health-related decisions, attempt to define the ways in which social and environmental factors influence these decisions and provide an insight into the dynamics influencing their behaviour.

Various models employed within the field of health promotion attempt to explain how individuals go about making health-related decisions. Among these are Becker's Health Belief Model 1984 (cited in Tones 1990) and the Fishbein and Ajzen's Theory of Reasoned Action 1980, 1985 (cited in Tones 1990). The Health Belief Model, according to Tones, highlights the role of four key beliefs in stimulating preventive health actions and it illustrates how the likelihood of action will be enhanced if the individual has a positive attitude to health and if some cue or trigger is provided. Therefore, the most important indicators of success are the four key beliefs, the number of preventive actions undertaken and the successful delivery of 'cues to action'.

Fishbein and Ajzen's 'Theory of Reasoned Action' separates beliefs from attitudes and emphasises the importance of 'significant others' on an individual's 'intention to act'. In doing these things, it improves on the Health Belief Model and allows for a more empirical approach. The often substantial gap between intention and practice is acknowledged and the relationship between beliefs, attitudes, normative factors, intention and practice are then expressible in mathematical terms.

However, even though both of these models are powerful, on their own they do not provide enough explanation of the issues involved in alcohol misuse, as they ignore the wider social and environmental factors which are known to be important in alcohol use. However, one model which has been applied to the prevention of alcohol and drug misuse is Tones' Health Action Model. That model demonstrates the importance of adopting a multifactorial strategy which embraces most specific approaches and incorporates the Health Belief Model, the Theory of Reasoned Action, and various other health-related theories. Therefore, it constitutes a sound basis for a theoretical framework when considering district alcohol strategies.

In his model, Tones (1990) suggests that there are a variety of factors which are directly or indirectly involved in alcohol misuse. A complex matrix of cultural, socio-economic, cognitive, affective, and psycho-social influences is involved, as can be seen in Figure 1 below. This can be used as a point of reference when discussing the relevance of the Health Action Model in helping to explain alcohol-related decision-making and for assisting in the process of devising interventions.

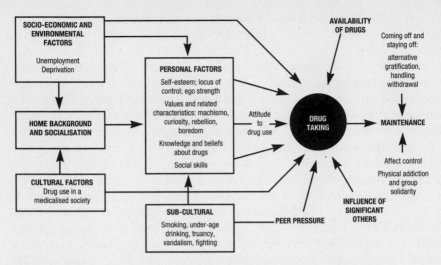

Figure 1 Misuse of drugs: psycho-social and environmental influences

According to Tones, the primary purpose of the model is to incorporate the major factors – environmental, interpersonal and intra-personal which influence individual decision-making and supply post-decisional support. Placing the major focus on education, it is also congruent with broader health promotion approaches. Additionally, and unlike other models, it indicates how 'healthy public policy' may be an essential prerequisite in 'making the healthy choice the easy choice'.

The Health Action Model is concerned with the ways in which the interaction between cognitive factors (knowledge and beliefs), a 'motivation system' (consisting of values, attitudes and drives) and the pressures from social norms and significant others may combine to affect an individual's intention to act (behavioural intention). Tones also illustrates how it recognises the importance of other factors, such as the physical or social environment and the possession of relevant knowledge and skills, which may either facilitate or inhibit the translation of a behavioural intention into action.

The crucial notion of feedback is very important in this model. The effect of any decision taken by a person will make itself felt, either in the short or longer term, by affecting either the belief system, the motivation system or both and it is important to provide either environmental or social support once such a decision has been made. Of course, it is this which makes it central to the doctrine of health promotion and which argues that environmental circumstances should be so structured that the healthy choice is the easy choice. Thus, it can be seen how, by implementing an alcohol strategy, a district will be achieving exactly this.

As might well be anticipated, there is a poor correlation between attitude and practice, and this is well documented. However, Tones (1990) seeks to account for this discrepancy in the model by drawing attention to various potential barriers which he categorises as: environmental, lack of knowledge and a deficiency in necessary skills. Certain 'facilitating factors' should be supplied, according the Tones, in order to deal with these barriers in implementing health promotion programmes. A district alcohol strategy should achieve this very goal.

Therefore, the model provides an important operational framework when considering district alcohol strategies. Support for the implementation of district alcohol strategies is to be found with the Faculty of Public Medicine of The Royal College of Physicians (1991), and with the government, recommending that the development and regular review of such local strategies is the best way forward.

More importantly, from the theoretical and academic perspective, the development of district alcohol strategies is totally consistent with the general principle and holistic approach of health promotion, as discussed in these pages. This is particularly so with respect to the concepts of creating supportive environments and strengthening community action, as outlined in the Ottawa Charter (1986, cited in Green and Raeburn 1990).

Despite this general enthusiasm, however, information about the development, effectiveness and overall national progress of district alcohol strategies is scarce. Posner (1992) has undertaken some research into regional alcohol strategies and found varying degrees of success, but the benefits of district alcohol strategies remain inadequately reported and hence a degree of doubt about their value persists. In closing this chapter, though, we can say that it is clear from its foregoing pages that in terms of the prevention of alcohol misuse and health promotion, community approaches are currently giving the most hope as the way forward. Bennett (1994) argues that, while there is very little published evidence, multi-agency collaboration at a district level is seen as fundamentally important and the pooling of creative thinking and resources is more likely to generate effective local action than any other strategy. Now needed is further research to determine, firstly, the quality of the strategies and, secondly, just how successful district alcohol strategies are proving to be.

14

THE PROBLEM OF ASSESSING HEALTH PROMOTION INITIATIVES

Rendering health promotion accountable

We have indicated that the most obvious expression of health promotion is in empowerment and that empowerment is reflected in the elaboration of community responses of some sort. Obviously there is no merit in any of this unless:

1 it can be shown that community programmes have, in fact, arisen in this way;
2 such community programmes are susceptible to assessment;
3 a general strategy can be drawn up for evaluating community programmes and, in so doing, legitimising (or the reverse) health promotion itself.

The idea of initiating community programmes of one type or another with the aim of achieving specific health promotion objectives is now well established. Green and Raeburn (1990) usefully summarise many of these. Some specific community-based health promotion areas stand out as having been enormously successful. Consider the field of cancer screening. There really has been a debate in this area, not only about the efficacy of health promotion but even of screening itself in terms of the numbers of lives saved which would not have been saved without it. The consensus view now appears to be that health promotion initiatives around cancer screening does increase the percentage of women coming forward, for instance, for breast cancer screening (NCI Breast Cancer Screening Consortium 1990). Another high-profile area for this type of community advocacy involves coronary health. For instance, the work of Green and Richard (1993) and of Shea and Basch (1990) both recognise its legitimacy.

Mental health has caused particular anguish in the health promotion community. As recently as 1992, the present author was asked to give a talk to an RCN sponsored Mental Heath Care Workers Conference. He spoke on the topic 'Mental Health Promotion' and was astounded by the frequency with which the mental healthcare nurses raised the objection that one cannot (and sometimes 'should not') empower the mentally ill as they need to learn to do what they are told, not make a nuisance of themselves by deciding unilaterally how to look after themselves.

It is doubtful whether that comment would be made today. However, even as far back as 1991, De Renzo, Byer, Grady and others had declared the necessity of a proactive approach to mental health promotion.

One could enumerate other areas of concern which have adopted a community health promotion approach, e.g. smoking and the attendant risk factors (COMMIT Research Group 1995) and comprehensive multifactorial health promotion initiatives (Wagner *et al.* 1991).

The recency with which the whole idea of even attempting to render health promotion subject to outcome measurement has meant the 'ideologies' clustered around the various possible attitudes to it are still more well established than the actual attempts at empirical research about them.

On doing the literature review for this chapter (early in 1997), this author found that health promotion evaluation has, until now, attracted four categories of papers:

1   articles assuming that a given research decision will render a comprehensive assessment feasible at the end;
2   articles about ongoing projects and embodying tentative outcome analyses;
3   articles purporting to present final outcomes assessment;
4   articles considering the philosophical and epistemological problems attendant upon treating health promotion initiatives in this way.

Articles from the first category are somewhat rare and often reflect a complete naivety about the implications, as well as lacking critical rigour. Obviously the greater part of what we know about community health promotion programmes can be found in the second group of articles. These articles provide a rich source of data, documenting various aspects of community programming. Regrettably, because these findings do not arise from controlled experiments, the status of the findings is to be regarded as problematic. The third group of articles can be most deceptive because their confident use of targets and performance indicators, and other academic paraphernalia often associated with the market forces ideology, very much obscures the real issue. Can, in fact, health promotion criteria be objectified as commodities in the short term?

One is often left with the feeling, after reading such accounts, that the whole question of 'risk factors' (Susser 1975) has to be sidelined because it is outside of experimental control. This, of course, makes a nonsense of attempting such an analysis from that point of view, but others would see it as indicating that community health promotion is not effective. In this, it is instructive to recall that a similar methodological debate dogged analyses of the impact of pre-school enrichment programmes for children from deprived backgrounds in the 1960s (Douglas *et al.* 1971).

It is the author's purpose in this chapter to focus the reader's attention largely on the epistemological difficulties reflected in the fourth group of articles.

Is health promotion assessable?

Many in health promotion are tempted to adopt what this author refers to as an 'inspirational' or essentially 'religio-mystical' attitude to the subject to guard against the restrictive and insensitive intrusion of limited 'economic' measures. But if the reader reflects back on the issues dealt with in Chapter 1, it will surely be appreciated that a retreat from scientific rigour is no solution at all and would, with ample justification, eventually exclude health promotion from serious consideration altogether. On the contrary, attempts must be made to quantify and measure outcomes and health promotion can justify itself on such rational criteria, but only if they are epistemologically valid. Our concern must be to critically interpret the market forces models of assessment, with their necessarily foreshortened time-frames of reference. This point is very well made, in another context (reforms in the NHS), by Julian Hart (1994).

Basically, the problem centres on what might be termed the 'commodification of health'. The whole apparatus of analysis of economic activities, with its emphasis on targets, objectives, performance indicators, and the like, assumes the existence of a defined commodity. For instance, to paraphrase Benjamin Franklin's famous comment, if I am in the business of producing mouse-traps, I can keep an exact record of the number produced in each quarter, to whom they are sold, and, most critically, how many mice they kill. In all of this, there is no ambiguity whatever as to the purpose of my product nor how to know if that purpose is being met. Moreover, there is also no ambiguity about who the producers are and who are the consumers. For instance, the mice who are killed are not the consumers, but rather the people who buy the traps to kill the mice are the consumers. The mouse-trap is a produced commodity and all of the other measures flow clearly from that fact.

Thus, for market forces style analysis to work properly, we need a defined commodity. What is the commodity in healthcare? One could ask a very similar question about 'education'. If we say 'health', then the patient is a 'consumer' buying 'health' from the producer. Who is the producer? The NHS? The doctor? In fact, is the patient really the consumer? Surely the objective is to improve the health of the community, otherwise why have a Secretary of State for Health? In that case, the doctor could be regarded as the 'consumer' and the client becomes a 'producer' in that, by being socially responsible enough to go to the doctor when germ-ridden, he/she is 'providing' health (as a commodity) to the community. The problem becomes even more intractable if we look at the issue of measuring outcomes.

The effects of a citizen's interaction with the doctor or the NHS generally are not easily measured. The outcomes cannot be measured, except in *very* approximate terms, over time. Mouse-traps, by comparison, are appealing in their simplicity. The improved 'quality of life' brought about by a person not having to put up with a belly-ache may result in him or her doing something quite unexpected from which the whole society benefits (or the reverse, of course) in unpredictable ways.

All of this, then, is not a problem to be avoided by fleeing into mysticism, but a challenge to be faced by creative mathematicians and statisticians. The aim is that, by meaningfully measuring outcomes of community health promotion, we can render community health promotion more responsive to rational control and scientific analysis. It is these difficult philosophical issues which need to be confronted by the people involved in any given community health promotion initiative, and, clearly, this discussion has to take place *before* any action is undertaken. Short-term measurable 'actions' with short-term measurable 'outcomes' will always be a temptation, but cannot stand in for health promotion assessment.

Problems with assessing individual health promotion initiatives

There are two major and abiding problems which confront us when we try to assess health promotion:

1 There are a number of different definitions of health promotion and presumably they would not be different if they all met the same criteria.
2 Since health promotion involves empowerment, it is not a phenomenon fixed in one point in time, like a measles injection or an appendectomy, but is a continuous and developing process. Moreover, the process is aimed at a desired outcome (or series of desired outcomes) which equip the person to assume a greater command over his/her life. In that sense, even the outcome (or outcomes) is also a process. Therefore, assessment of the phenomenon, and how such an assessment is mediated, depends on whether one is evaluating:

   a   the process on its way to an outcome;
   b   the outcome (or one of the outcomes) as an end point;
   c   the outcome (or one of the outcomes) as a process in enhancing the person's life.

Let us consider these problems. Although the fact is that there are several different definitions of health promotion, further analysis reveals that most of these differences are differences in degree rather than of kind. That does not trivialise the problem, but it allows us to tie it in with the 'process/outcome' problem and often to resolve it in the context of resolving that one. With respect to that second problem, Kickbusch (1994) incorporates the primacy of 'process' into her definition of health promotion: 'Health promotion is a process for initiative, managing and implementing change . . . . a process of personal, organisational and policy development'.

Another approach to untangling the semantic difficulties posed by all of this is to try to differentiate between 'terminal' and 'instrumental' values (Rokeach 1983). His approach involves dividing up the objectives of any health promotion initiative into two categories:

1   instrumental objectives;
2   terminal goals.

Instrumental objectives, as the name suggests, denotes the short-term aims, attainment of which are intended to move the long-term process of health promotion initiative one step further forward. For instance, let us take an unusually dramatic example. A person diagnosed as a paranoid schizophrenic and living out on the street, might, as part of a process of empowerment, so order his/her life sufficiently to take appropriate medication at the right times. That in itself no doubt was one of the short-term objectives in the mediation of an entire long-term health promotion programme.

Terminal goals obviously refer to the 'end-state' of the enterprise. These are the long-term goals which hierarchise and lend purpose to all of the instrumental objectives. The long-term goal might itself be comparatively modest. For instance, for the schizophrenic it might not be recovery from the condition, but to learn to live with it so that it intrudes as minimally as possible on his/her life and on the lives of people in the community of which he/she is a member. For instance, to be able to behave reasonably predictably, to attend out-patient clinics as required, to keep clean, perhaps to gain employment, might represent the acme of health promotion for that person in that situation.

Usually, of course, the entire health promotion initiative is itself less spectacular and more easily divided into instrumental objectives and terminal goals. In Chapters 12 and 13, for instance, we considered some of the health promotion aspects of tobacco and alcohol use. Probably most readers of this book have had some experience with one or other of these extremely common health promotion problems and can easily make a list for one or another of them of instrumental objectives and terminal goals.

Establishing a framework for assessment

Obviously health promotion initiatives, be they modest and common or more esoteric and directed at what appear to be much rarer and intractable problems, involve outlays of capital, labour and other resources. They commit both the individual and the community to an enterprise in which great expectations attach to the outcome. This involves a high element of

---

Chart A

Definitions of health promotion

- a strategy 'aimed at informing, influencing and assisting both individuals and organisations so that they will accept more responsibility and be more active in matters affecting mental and physical health' (Lalonde 1974)
- 'seeks the development of community and individual measures which can help [people] to develop lifestyles that can maintain and enhance the state of well-being' (US Department of Health, Education and Welfare 1979)
- 'any combination of health education and related organisational, political and economic interventions designed to facilitate behavioural and environmental adaptations that will improve or protect health'(Green 1980)
- 'the process of enabling people to increase control over, and to improve their health' (WHO 1984, 1987; Epp 1986)
- 'the maintenance and enhancement of existing levels of health through the implementation of effective programs, services, and policies'(Goodstadt et al. 1987)
- 'the science and art of helping people choose their lifestyles to move toward a state of optimal health' (O'Donnell 1989)
- 'the process of enabling individuals and communities to increase control over the determinants of health and thereby improve their health' (Stachechenko and Jenicek 1990)
- 'efforts through the overlapping spheres of health education, prevention and health protection to enhance positive health and prevent ill-health' (Downie et al. 1990)
- 'any activity or program designed to improve social and environmental living conditions such that people's experience of well-being is increased'(Labonte and Little 1992)
- 'any combination of educational, organizational, economic, and environmental supports for conditions of living and behaviour of individuals, groups or communities conducive to health' (Green and Ottoson 1994)

---

trust on the part of those who pay the bills (e.g. tax-payers), work in the enterprise (e.g. health visitors) and people to whom the initiative is directed. This element of trust is pivotal and must be sustained. One way of expediting its survival is to organise such transparent systems so that they are readily accountable to all of the participants mentioned.

Part of this objective is met by specifying ahead of time what the short- and long-term objectives are, estimates of the length of time required to achieve each, etc. But to do that, the health promoters have to be clear as to which definition of health promotion they are using. Once this is clear, the definition used must be deconstructed so as to be able to objectively and empirically recognise and measure the extent to which the separate criteria of the definition used are being satisfied by the manner in which the initiative is being mediated (Potvin and Macdonald 1995; Rootman and Raeburn 1994; Springett *et al.* 1995). These same authors, along with Goodstadt *et al.* (1987), have arrived at a set of definitions (see Chart A) which can be deconstructed in terms of four criteria, as follows:

1   terminal goals;
2   instrumental objectives;
3   instrumental processes;
4   instrumental action.

Epistemological problems with the taxonomy

We live in the age of the flow-chart, an age when complex ideas and philosophical ambiguity can be made plain by displaying a few boxes, triangles, circles, etc., cunningly labelled, and with arrows busily darting back and forth across the page between them. In this author's jaundiced view, this sort of thing is sometimes used as a substitute for the austere and reasoned discourse of conventional scholarship. Without labouring that point unnecessarily, health promotion seems to attract more than its fair share of this kind of 'sociological wired-up geometry'. The problems arise, of course, as soon as one stops considering the paradigm in question as a nicely dove-tailed piece of theory and tries to apply it.

The foregoing taxonomy does not fall into this category because it is intellectually honest, but it still requires considerable epistemological analysis before it can be used. The basic problem is the aforementioned one of definition – in any given case, are we speaking of a generally health-consciousness enhancing process, or the end-point of such a process, or the manner in which such an end-point can enhance the rest of one's life? However, the logistics of the situation are, in fact, more situation-specific and less wide open than such comments may suggest. Instrumental objectives readily fall into one of two categories:

1   a category targeted on the environment, as in making reference to the material context in which the person has to live his/her life;
2   a category aimed at the role of the individual person, as in considering new and healthier lifestyles.

These have each attracted insightful research and commentary. Thus, with respect to the environmental aspect, one should consider the work of Labonte and Little (1992), while with respect to personal and psychological growth, one might with profit look at the work of O'Donnell (1989). In some of the definitions, it is rather difficult to identify the processes to which reference is made. Lalonde's definition avoids that problem by specifying the process as being able to 'accept more responsibility and to be more active'. Likewise, the WHO definition designates the process as one of 'increasing control'. Most of the other definitions in Chart A do not so cogently identify the relevant processes on which presumably they are based.

The working health promoter, of course, has to arrive at his or her own working definition of what initiatives, from which there are always so many to choose, he/she will accept as constituting 'health promotion' for the purpose of in-process assessment. This, of course, is not to say that initiatives not classifiable as 'health promotion' are any less worthy. All it is saying is that one is not assessing them as health promotion and therefore cannot render a judgement on their relative merit. Throughout this book, the author's overriding criterion as to whether an initiative is health promotion or not hinges on the operational scope accorded the process of empowerment. For instance, screening programmes do not necessarily 'empower' (in fact, they often disempower) and the same can be said for many preventive health programmes.

Assessment of health promotion initiatives has to be taken seriously if for no other reason than that it has to provide managers and like-minded people with a justification for funding the projects in question. Therefore, it is crucial that the health promoter focus on initiatives which do meet the empowerment criterion and which can therefore be classified as health promotion.

In bringing this book to an end, then, let us consider what we shall mean when we speak of 'assessing' or 'evaluating' health promotion.

Defining and interpreting assessment

Probably the discipline most familiar with the problems associated with assessment is education, but, especially since the 1960s, a number of other areas have had to engage with it, including occupational psychology, aptitude, personnel management, etc. Until fairly recently educational assessment had concentrated exclusively on ascertaining how well (or badly) individual people coped with set tasks. The idea of assessing programmes and/or procedures, rather than people, is a relatively new one. When this sort of thing was first attempted, educational theorists were convinced that educational techniques could be empirically assessed with respect to one another on purely objective grounds. Of course, such an optimistic view assumed that 'teaching' was some sort of a science and could be assessed and measured independently of the subject matter to which it was applied, the people receiving the instruction, the personal values of the teacher, etc.

This view of the structure of the teaching–learning process led to the enunciating of the ideal of 'value-free teaching'. Very quickly it was realised that even to attempt value-free learning and teaching would be tantamount to producing rapidly comfortable programmes with little engagement of imagination or passion (Scriven 1973). But, as well, education as a discipline has conferred on the process of evaluation some extremely useful techniques, such as summative evaluation and formative evaluation, i.e. the question of precisely measuring outcomes when they present and also while in the process of being realised.

An increasing preoccupation with the financial outlays required to run various programmes has lent an urgency to evaluation and has created the need to engage in it as impartially as possible. Healthcare, being as expensive as it is, was one of the first areas to be targeted with a view to isolating effective models and effective criteria for assessment. With its emphasis on the less tangible attributes of empowerment, health promotion has attracted considerable interest. The best theoretical protocol for assessing health promotion initiatives is developed by Rootman, Goodstadt, Potvin and Springett in an as yet unpublished work.

They argue that five issues delineate a framework for evaluating health promotion, namely:

1   social programming;
2   knowledge construction;
3   valuing;
4   knowledge use;
5   evaluation procedures.

These can each be elaborated and targeted at health promotion, as follows:

Social programming

Any health promotion initiative, be it for an individual or for an entire community, has a specific and definable aim. It is itself made up of a series of assessable components. For example, *process evaluation* (Rossi and Freeman 1989) is directed at resources and procedures, while *outcome evaluating* deals with the changing interplay between procedures and resources while the target problem is being addressed. In theory, this means that the relationship between the programme and its target can be expressed in such a way that proximal, intermediate and distal outcomes can be identified first and then assessed to ascertain if the programme is internally consistent. Green and Kreuter (1991) produced such a model for health promotion and called it the PRECEDE/PROCEED Model. The PRECEDE component consists of each of the educational, environmental, epidemiological and organisational diagnoses. But each of these then corresponds to defining outcome indicators and these constitute the PROCEED component.

Knowledge construction

This attribute has been the subject of intense philosophical debate, most of it centred on the epistemological difficulties arising from treating programmes as 'natural phenomena' to which reductionist techniques of analysis can be applied. But, as with attempts at 'value-free' education, it is now generally agreed that it is unrealistic to posit the existence of a neutral observer to referee the process. This is particularly the case in an intensely 'people sensitive' area such as health promotion, in which the goal of empowerment requires acknowledgement by all concerned of so many intangibles.

Cook (1985) suggested a position midway between neutral empiricism and inchoate value-intensity. This involves a high degree of eclecticism and the recognition of introspective reaction. For instance, consider the difficulty with alcohol programmes in the community or the problems recognisable as an amalgam of racial marginalisation, adolescence and sickle-cell disease. Cook's approach has been criticised because it is compelled to draw from several disciplines. However, this is a strength when applied to health promotion.

Valuing

The purpose of any assessment, of course, ultimately is about designating a programme as having a particular 'value'. There are various approaches to the valuing, all belonging to one of two principal categories – prescriptive or descriptive. Prescriptive approaches designate certain desirable attributes, tolerance, economic equity, human dignity, etc., against which the legitimacy of programmes can be tested. Descriptive approaches, on the other hand, refer to the values agenda elaborated by the participants in the programme, be it one person or many. It is their values that are then used to assess the efficacy of the programmes.

This fits in perfectly with the goals of empowerment and neighbourhood advocacy in health promotion.

Knowledge use

Information gathered over the life of any given health promotion initiative for use in then evaluating its effectiveness is, of course, itself part of the knowledge package associated with that programme. Rossi and Freeman (1989) recognise three possible uses of this accumulating knowledge base:

1 instrumental use;
2 conceptual use;
3 persuasive use.

Instrumental use of assessment measures is enhanced through ascertaining who the likely users will be, communicating with them frequently about what they anticipate from their participation in the initiative and conferring as much control as possible to the users.

Conceptual use involves encouraging the participants to extrapolate from the assessment results sufficiently to think more generally and globally about the issue raised. To give an example, a single-mothers' group with which this author worked in Tower Hamlets soon moved from the specifics of their own primary aged children's problems to the general issue of the role of the home in promoting facility with the basic skills of literacy and numeracy in school.

Persuasive use involves basing user advocacy of the programme outside of the group on the assessment already carried out. In other words, this introduces an element of 'teacher training' or 'public speaking instruction', a vital element in developing the assertiveness that one has a right to associate with empowerment.

Evaluation procedures

This general area embraces a host of broadly logistic questions, such as: Is an empirical assessment necessary? For what would the information so obtained be used? How can such an assessment be made without distorting the original aims of the health promotion initiative concerned? Considerable theoretical work has been done on these issues by Shadish et al. (1991). They promote the view that an effective evaluation procedure makes clear what losses and gains attach to the integrity of the programme from each aspect of assessment.

There is some disagreement about when such questions should be asked. Patton (1982) advocates such a high level of frequency of communication between the health promoters and the participant that change in assessment policy can be made day-to-day, whereas Campbell and Stanley (1963) take the line that the assessors should have only minimal contact with the users in order to enhance the objectivity of the former's findings. Nutbeam et al.

190

(1990) advocate a policy of close collaboration between programme managers and users during the various 'departmental' or 'process' assessments but an increasing level of separation as the programme moves on to a dissemination phase.

Conceptualising the role of assessment in health promotion

Assessment of health promotion initiatives is important for a host of good, practical reasons. Not the least of these is the fact that the stated and implied aims of such initiatives are often so nebulous that it is even difficult to arrive at a coherent method for distinguishing between improvements that were already 'on the way' implicitly in the dynamics of the enterprise before the proposed initiative was implemented, from those that were definitely brought about by the initiative. This is not said in criticism of health promotion as being 'good-hearted fuzziness' or a rag-bag of clichés and 'motherhood statements'. Rather it recognises that, since health promotion has to recognise the cruciality of the participatory element at all stages and the autonomy of the participants, it finds it hard to lay out an easily assessed programme that, say, a prospective funder can validate.

Increasingly, therefore, health promoters find themselves on a search for 'programme assessment models' or 'evaluation strategy models' that are anchored in academic acceptance and are practical enough to persuade funders and yet can be conveniently applied to health promotion. Satisfying the first two criteria is no problem. In the last decade dozens of evaluation models have been put forward and have been incorporated into the academic realm of acceptance. For instance, see the 1996 publication *Empowerment Evaluation – Knowledge and Tools for Self-Assessment and Accountability* by Fetterman *et al*. It is a compendium.

But the existence of a plethora of models does not meet our needs in itself. It is their applicability to health promotion which is the problem. The issue here is to pin-point with some degree of precision the actual issues that render health promotion so difficult to assess. This author suggests that there are three:

1   maintaining participation at all levels;
2   respecting the integrity of individual empowerment;
3   being able to separate 'outcomes' from 'processes' and from extraneous development unrelated to the initiative concerned.

Once we establish those as criteria, the vast literature of 'evaluation/ assessment' can be narrowed down drastically. In Britain some of the best work in this area, without doubt, is being done at the Institute for Health at Liverpool John Moore's University under Jane Springett and Linda Gibson. In North America, Canada seems to retain its dominant position in modern health promotion – in the tradition of one of its leading originators, Marc Lalonde – and, in the particular topic of evaluation of health promotion initiatives, the work of Rootman, Goodstadt and Potvin stand out.

The three aforementioned criteria are all, of course, heavily contextualised, both institutionally and at the level of individual experience. It therefore becomes necessary to find some way of unravelling these extraneous issues before evaluation procedures can even be planned. In 1995, a most useful paper on this very topic was produced (Springett *et al.*) and much is to be gained from reading it.

Contextual problems

For instance, of all the theories in health promotion, how can one know which is applicable to the evaluation of a given programme? In this, health promotion theorists find themselves in a position very similar to that of Von Helmholz who, in the late nineteenth century, and inspired by the success of good models (e.g. Darwin's theory of evolution, through the twin processes of natural selection and reproductive isolation, made a particular impact on him), was determined to come up with a 'theory of everything' (TOE) – a sort of unified field theory that would usefully model and predict scientific insight. Although Von Helmholz never did find his TOE, there are two points that health promotion needs to remember:

1 Von Helmholz's failure on that undertaking did not stop him from making other smaller-scale, but useful, contributions to science.
2 It did not stop other people from looking for a TOE and, indeed, Stephen Hawkins is still hard at it.

An attempt has been made to develop an inclusive theory of health promotion (Martin and McQueen 1989), in the hope that once such a model was in place, evaluation procedures could be rendered unambiguous with respect to it. As we know, Martin and McQueen did not achieve their aim, but we still must assess what we do. That brings us to the problem of methodology.

It has been said that the American Evaluation Association recognises about 150 programme assessment strategies. Of course, most of them are thankfully not applicable to health promotion, but it still leaves us with a lot of work to do. The problem is rendered more obscure in health promotion because of the involvement, dictated by neighbourhood advocacy, with impinging community values which restrict solutions but are not themselves part of the problem. For instance, ethical issues in health promotion are often different from ethical issues implicit in a project's impact on some other aspect of community life.

In any health promotion initiative, the aims have social and political implications. There is little room for 'studied neutrality' here, for the aims have to satisfy a defined set of objectives which are bound to be at variance with some other political initiative. Often the aims addressed by the health promotion initiative are in the interest of the relatively *powerless*, because this is an objective of empowerment – whereas most existing political structures are designed to meet the needs of the already *powerful*. For that reason, any attempt at assessing or evaluating the effectiveness of a given health promotion initiative has to be fully cognisant of the politics of the context. One must adjust to prevailing attitudes to a large extent, rather than try to change them.

Any change of powerful attitudes should, according to health promotion theory, come about through the efforts of people empowered by the initiative and not as one of the aims of the initiative itself.

Again, this raises even more immediate problems. In any initiative, a variety of categories of people are involved: consumers, health promoters, healthcare workers, funders and even the people assessing the programme. In certain non-health promotion contexts it is a fairly straightforward problem to identify the roles of these categories and to hierarchise them. But in health promotion, participation is a key theme and this renders the issues much more complex. Participation demands not only that each of the categories has an input, but that each is satisfied that the input concerned is accorded appropriate weight in decision-making. That is one reason why an important component in the academic preparation of health promoters is training in group dynamics and interpersonal skills.

All of the foregoing implies the need for a high degree of psychological and intellectual flexibility on the part of all of the people involved, not only the health promoters themselves. For instance, fundholders demand specific answers that can be used for quality control and for audit purposes. If they were not aware of the fact before, they very quickly find out that the criteria useful for audit and quality control in the production and marketing of mouse-traps do not work so well in evaluating health promotion initiatives.

In 1964 the present author was involved in an adult literacy programme as part of President Johnson's 'War on Poverty' in an economically deprived area of California. He was very fortunate in securing the services of a cost accountant, for audit and quality control purposes, who also had Bata Shoes as one of his clients. As our project drew to a close, the author thanked the accountant and asked him if he had found the experience interesting. His reply clearly underlined the problem referred to above. He said: 'Interesting? You bet! It was exhilarating and frightening, like trying to corner a rat and then realising that the rat was really a grizzly bear and he was cornering you! I'm really glad I had this experience, but I'll feel safer when I'm back with shoes!'

The imperative of participation

Spingett *et al.*, in their aforementioned 1995 paper, recognise that the key difficulty is that imposed by the philosophical imperative of participation. They argue that participation does clarify what exactly the categories of people are, or as they say, who the 'stakeholders' are. It makes their relative hold on 'power' clear as well and allows them to define, from their own perspective, what they see as the role of the assessment. This, in turn, leads to a general modification across all of the categories, of stated aims, criteria for quality control and means of assessment.

Their evaluation framework is predicated on six broad attitudinal foci, as follows:

1   It has to be recognised as broadly applicable to the theory of evaluation generally, to confer academic credibility in it, but also to be specifically relevant to the particular initiative at which it will be targeted.
2   It has to demonstrate that it is philosophically consistent with health promotion ideals – e.g. intended to *empower* rather than *direct*.
3   It has to reflect a concern for translating the empowerment of individuals into action at the neighbourhood level and, beyond the level of neighbourhood advocacy, to the more politically problematic area of community intersectorality.
4   It has to demonstrate that it is flexible enough to respond to changes in contextual community variables as they impinge on the initiative in question.
5   It has to be inclusive enough to monitor every stage from the setting of the agenda to the collating and interpretation of the outcomes.
6   It should be transparently and equally communicating to all of the stakeholders' interests.

It is this author's view that the elaboration of evaluation frameworks along these, or similar, lines is the next major step to be taken in establishing the relevance and potency of the health promotion concept as a force for progress towards health for all in the individual, the community and the world. May it engage our best minds and our most innovatory actionists.

REFERENCES

Chapter 1

Banks, A.L and Hislop, J.A (1962) *Health and Hygiene*, 2nd edn, Cambridge: Cambridge University Press.

Barrett, D. (1964) *Aristophanes*, trans., Harmondsworth: Penguin.

Bellamy, D. and Pfister, D. (1992) *World Medicine*, Oxford: Blackwell.

Daremberg, C. (1895) *La Médecine Dans Homère*, Paris: Maison Hachette.

Dubos, R. (1995) 'Mirage of Health', in B. Davey, A. Grays and C. Seale (eds), *Health and Disease: A Reader*, 2nd edn, Buckingham: Open University Press, pp. 4–10.

Farrington, B. (1949) *Green Science and Its Meaning for Us*, Harmondsworth: Penguin.

Illich, I. (1975) *Medical Nemesis*, part 1, London: Calder and Boyers.

Jones, G. and Washington, A. (1926) *Hippocrates*, trans., Cambridge, MA: Loeb Classical Library.

Jones, W. (1945) *Hippocrates and the Corpus Hippocraticum*, Oxford: Oxford University Press, vol. 3, pp. 192–219, vol. 7, p. 388.

Kassebaum, G. and Baumann, B. (1965) 'Dimensions of the Sick Role in Chronic Illness', *Journal of Health & Social Behaviour* 6: 16–27

Lalonde, M. (1974) *A New Perspective on the Health of Canadians*, Ottawa: Information Canada.

Larkey, S. (1936) 'The Hippocratic Oath in Elizabethan England', *Bulletin of the History of Medicine* 4: 201–219.

MacDonald, T. (1994) 'A Semantic Analysis of Health Promotion', *British Osteopathic Journal* XIV: 30–39.

McKeown, T. (1979) *The Role of Medicine*, Oxford: Blackwell.

Navarro, V. (1980) 'Work, Ideology and Science: The Case of Medicine', *Social Science and Medicine* 14: 191–205.

Radice, B. (1973) *Who's Who in the Ancient World*, Harmondsworth: Penguin.

Singer, C., Underwood, C. and Underwood, E.A. (1962) *A Short History of Medicine*, Oxford: Clarendon Press, pp. 346–348.

Waldron, H.A. (1978) *The Medical Role in Environmental Health*, Oxford: Oxford University Press.

Walker, M. (1930) *Pioneers in Public Health*, Edinburgh: Edinburgh University Press.

Woodham-Smith, C. (1991) *The Reason Why*, Harmondsworth: Penguin, pp. 128–143.

Chapter 2

Basaglia, F.O. (1986) 'The Changing Culture of Health and the Difficulties of Public Health to Cope with It', *Vienna Dialogue on Health Policy and Health Promotion – Towards a New Conception of Public Health, European Social Development Programme*, no. 81, Brussels: EEC Publications.

Bunton, R. and Macdonald, G. (1992) *Health Promotion: Disciplines and Diversity*, London: Routledge.

Engel, G. (1989) 'The Need for a New Medical Model – A Challenge for Biomedical Science', *Holistic Medicine* 4 (1): 17–21.

Gardner, M. (1991) *The New Age: Notes of a Fringe Watcher*, New York: Prometheus Books.

Hibbert, C. (1989) *The English: A Social History 1066–1945*, London: Guild Publishing.

Lalonde, M. (1974) *A New Perspective on the Health of Canadians*, Ottawa: Information Canada.

Lovelock, J. (1979) *Gaia: A New Look at Life on Earth*, Oxford: Oxford University Press.

MacDonald, T. (1984) *Peace Studies in the Primary School: Education*, vol. 2, Sydney: New South Wales Department of Education, pp. 29–44.

—— (1994) 'Health Promotion: A Semantic Analysis' *British Journal of Osteopathy* 4: 14–21.

Oakley, A. (1980) *Women Confined: Towards a Sociology of Childbirth*, Oxford: Martin Robertson.

Parsons, T. (1969) *The Social System*, London: Routledge & Kegan Paul.

Prescott, R. (1991) 'The Impact of Environmental Education on Inner-City Children', *Primary Education* 4: 125–129.

Rosenstock, I. (1974) 'Historical Origins of the Health Belief Model', *Health Education Monographs* 2: 409–419.

Sayers, J. (1982) *Biological Politics: Feminist and Anti-Feminist Perspectives*, London: Tavistock.

Shapere, D. (1977) 'Scientific Theories and Their Domains', in F. Suppe (ed.), *The Structure of Scientific Theories*, Urbana, IL: University of Illinois Press.

Tones, K. (1992) *Empowerment, Control and the Promotion of Health*, Melbourne: Deakin University Press.

Turner, B. (1990) 'The Interdisciplinary Curriculum: From Social Medicine to Postmodernism', *Sociology of Health and Illness* 12 (1): 241–248.

WHO (1977) *Alma Ata Declaration*, no. 6, Copenhagen: WHO.

Zola, I. (1975) 'In the Name of Health and Illness', *Social Science and Medicine* 9: 183–188.

Chapter 3

Basaglia, F.O. (1986) 'The Changing Culture of Health and the Difficulties of Public Health to Cope with It', *Vienna Dialogue on Health Policy and Health Promotion – Towards a New Conception of Public Health, European Social Development Programme*, no. 81, Brussels: EEC Publications.

REFERENCES

Brubaker, B.H. (1983) 'Health Promotion a Linguistic Analysis', *Advances in Nursing Science* 5 (3): 1–14.

Chalmers, K. and Farrell, P. (1983) 'Nursing Interventions for Health Promoting', *Nurse Practitioner* 8 (10): 62.

Chave, S.P. (1986) 'The Origins and Development of Public Health', *Oxford Textbook of Public Health*, Vol. 1, Milton Keynes: Open University Press.

Clarke, J.N. (1992) 'Feminist Methods in Health Promotion Research, *Canadian Journal of Public Health* 83 (suppl. 1): 54–57.

DHSS (1981) *Primary Health Care in Inner London* (Acheson Report), London: HMSO.

Doucette, S. (1989) 'The Changing Role of Nurses: the Perspective of the Medical Services Branch', *Canadian Journal of Public Health* 80 (2): 92–94.

Duffy, M.E. (1988) 'Health Promotion in the Family: Current Findings and Directives for Nursing Research', *Journey of Advanced Nursing* 13 (1): 109–117.

Dunn, H.L. (1959) 'High-levels, Wellness in Man and Society', *American Journal of Public Health* 49: 786.

Epp, J. (1986) 'Achieving Health for All: A Framework for Health Promotion', *Canadian Journal of Public Health* 77 (6): 393–430.

Ewles, L. and Simnett, L. (1985) *Promoting Health: A Practical Guide*, 1st edn, London: Scutari Press.

Green, L.W. and Anderson, C.L. (1986) *Community Health*, 5th edn, St Louis, MO: Mosby.

Hammond, A. (1950) *The Urban Poor*, Manchester: Gollancz.

Hart, J. (1988) *A New Kind of Doctor*, London: Merlin.

Hayman, H.S. (1965) 'An Ecological View of Health and Health Education', *Journal of School Health* 35 (3): 48–58.

Lalonde, M. (1974) *A New Perspective on the Health of Canadians*, Ottawa: Information Canada.

Little, C. (1992) 'Health for All by the Year 2000: Where is it Now?', *Nursing and Healthcare* 13: 198–201.

Maslow, A. (1954) *Motivation and Personality*, New York: Harper & Row.

Parish, R. and Root, D. (1991) *Methods for Evaluating Health Education Programs*, Toronto, Ont.: University of Toronto Press.

Parsons, T. (1972) 'Definitions of Health and Illness in the Light of American Values and Societal Structure', in E. Jaco and R. Garthy (eds), *Patients, Physicians and Illness*, Glencoe, IL: Free Press.

Raeburn, J. (1992) 'Health Promotion Research with Courtesy: Keeping a People Perspective' *Canadian Journal of Public Health* 83: 20–24.

Shaver, J.F. (1985) 'A Biopsychosocial View of Human Health', *Nursing Outlook* 33: 186–191.

Simard, L. (1992) *A Saskatchewan Vision for Health: A Framework for Change*, Regina, Sask.: Saskatchewan Health.

Tannahill, A. (1985) 'What is Health Promotion?', *Health Education Journal* 44: 21–29.

Townsend, E.A. (1992) 'Institutional Ethnography: Explicating the Social Organisation of Professional Health Practices Intending Client Empowerment', *Canadian Journal of Public Health* 83 (suppl. 1): 558–561.

Whitehead, M. (1982) *The Health Divide: Inequalities in Health in the 1980s*, London: Health Education Council.

WHO (1946) *Constitution of the World Health Organisation*, first principle, New York: WHO.

—— (1977) *Alma Ata Declaration*, no. 6, Copenhagen: WHO.

—— (1978) *Primary Healthcare: Report of the International Conference on Primary Healthcare at Alma-Ata, USSR, September 6–12*, Geneva: WHO/UNICEF.

—— (1984) *Health Promotion: A Discussion Document on the Concepts and Principles*, Copenhagen: WHO.

—— (1986) *Health Promotion Concepts and Principles in Action: A Policy Framework*, Copenhagen: WHO.

Zinssner, A. (1952) *Rats, Lice and History*, Boston, MA: Houghton-Mifflin.

Chapter 4

Airhihenbuwa, C.O. (1993) 'Health Promotion for Child Survival in Africa: Implications for Cultural Appropriateness', *International Journal of Health Education* 12: 10–15.

—— (1994) 'Health Promotion and the Discourse in Culture: Implications for Empowerment', *Health Education Quarterly* 21 (3): 345–353.

Akin-Ojundeji, O. (1991) 'Asserting Psychology in Africa', *The Psychologist: Bulletin of the British Psychological Society* 4 (1): 2–4.

Antaki, C. (1989) 'Social Psychology in Nicaragua', *The British Psychological Society, Social Psychology Section Newsletter* 21: 32.

Berry, J. (1969) 'On Cross-cultural Compatibility', *International Journal of Psychology* 4: 119–128.

Davies, S. (1993) 'Psychology in Agony: Letter to the Bulletin of the British Psychological Society', *The Psychologist: Bulletin of the British Psychological Society* June: 249.

Foster, D. and Low-Potgieter, J. (eds) (1991) *Social Psychology in South Africa*, Johannesburg: Lexicon Publishers.

Freud, S. (1953) 'The Future Prospects of Psychoanalytic Therapy', in *Complete Works of Sigmund Freud*, vol. 11, London: Hogarth Press.

—— (1984a) *Beyond the Pleasure Principle*, Harmondsworth: Penguin.

—— (1984b) *The Ego and the Id*, Harmondsworth: Penguin.

—— (1991a) *The Interpretation of Dreams*, Harmondsworth: Penguin.

—— (1991b) *Sigmund Freud: On Sexuality*, vol. 7, Harmondsworth: Penguin.

Harris, A. (1990) 'A Psychologist in El Salvador', *The Psychologist: Bulletin of the British Psychological Society* 3 (6): 264–266.

Jahoda, G. (1983) 'Has Social Psychology a Distinctive Contribution to Make?' in P. Blackler (ed.), *Social Psychology in Developing Countries*, Chichester: Wiley.

Lalonde, M. (1974) *A New Perspective on the Health of Canadians*, Ottawa: Information Canada.

Letlake-Rennery, K. (1993) 'Psychology in South Africa', *The Psychologist: Bulletin of the British Psychological Society* April: 168.

MacDonald, T. (1983) *Perspectives on Illiteracy*, Newcastle, Australia: Newcastle University Press.

—— (1996) 'Global Health Promotion: Challenge to a Eurocentric Concept?', *British Journal of Therapy and Rehabilitation* 3 (5): 279–283.

Masson, J. (1992) *Against Therapy*, London: Fontana.

Omari, I. (1983) 'The Application of Social Psychology in Developing Countries', in P. Blackler (ed.), *Social Psychology in Developing Countries*, Chichester: Wiley.

Pike, K.L. (1966) *Language in Relation to a United Theory of the Structure of Human Behaviour*, The Hague: Mouton.

Reeler, A. (1991) 'Psychological Disorders in Primary Care and the Development of Clinical Services: An African Perspective', *The Psychologist: Bulletin of the British Psychological Society* 4: 349–353.

Riger, S. (1993) 'What's Wrong with Empowerment?', *American Journal of Community Psychology* 21 (3): 279–292.

Sinha, D. (1983) 'Applied Social Psychology and Problems of National Development', in P. Blackler (ed.), *Social Psychology in Developing Countries*, Chichester: Wiley.

Smith, P. (1991/2) 'Does Social Psychology Travel Well?' *The British Psychological Society: Social Psychology Section Newsletter* 26: 41–52.

Sophocles (1924) *Oedipus Rex*, trans. B.B. Rogers, Cambridge, MA: Loeb Classical Library.

Tembo, K. (1991) 'Evaluation of Source of Messages on AIDS by College Students', *Malawi Medical Journal* 7 (3): 117–118.

Chapter 5

Alaszewski, A. (1995) 'Restructuring Health and Welfare Professions in the UK: the Impact of Internal Markets on the Medical, Nursing and Social Work Professions', in T. Johnson, G. Larkin and M. Saks (eds), *Health Professions and the State in Europe*, London: Routledge.

Allsop, J. (1995) 'Shifting Spheres of Opportunity: the Processional Powers of General Practitioners within the British National Health Service', in T. Johnson, G. Larkin and M. Saks (eds), *Health Professions and the State in Europe*, London: Routledge.

Baum, F. and Saunders, D. (1995) 'Can Health Promotion and Primary Health Care Achieve Health for All without a Return to their more Radical Agenda?', *Health Promotion International* 10 (2): 149–160.

Butler, P. (1996) 'Against the Grain', *Health Service Journal* 106 (5532): 12.

Calnan, M. and Williams, S. (1995) 'Challenges to Professional Autonomy in the United Kingdom? The Perceptions of General Practitioners', *International Journal of Health Services* 25 (2): 219–241.

Calnan, M., Boulton, M. and Williams, A. (1986) 'Health Education and General Practitioners: a Critical Appraisal', in S. Rodmell and A. Watt (eds), *The Politics of Health Education: Raising the Issues*, London: Routledge.

Caraher, M. (1994) 'A Sociological Approach to Health Promotion for Nurses in an Institutional Setting', *Journal of Advanced Nursing* 20: 544–551.

Catford, J. (1995) 'Health Promotion in the Market Place: Constraints and Opportunities', *Health Promotion International* 10 (1): 41–21.

Cole, A. (1996) 'Opportunity Knocks', *Health Visitor* 69 (12): 484–485.

Cook, R. (1995) 'Health Promotion in the Primary Care Setting', *Health Visitor* 68 (6): 289–290.

Cowley, S. (1995) 'Health Promotion in the General Practice Setting', *Health Visitor* 68 (5): 199–201.

Cox, C. and Mead, A. (eds) (1975) *A Sociology of Medical Practice,* Gateshead: Collier-Macmillan.

Donaldson, R.J. and Donaldson, L.J. (1993) *Essential Public Health Medicine,* Lancaster: Kluwer.

Draper, P. (1991) *Health through Public Policy*, London: Green Print.

Farrant, W. (1991) 'Addressing the Contradictions: Health Promotion and Community Health Action in the United Kingdom', *International Journal of Health Services* 21 (3): 423–439.

Freidson, E. (1970) *Professional Dominance,* Chicago, IL: Atherton Press

Gill, D. (1975) 'The British National Health Service: Professional Determinants of Administrative Structure', in C. Cox and A. Mead (eds), *A Sociology of Medical Practice*, Gateshead: Collier-Macmillan.

Illich, I. (1979) *Limits to Medicine: Medical Nemesis: the Expropriation of Health*, Harmondsworth: Penguin.

Johnson, T., Larkin, G. and Saks, M. (eds) (1995) *Health Professions and the State in Europe*, London: Routledge.

Jones, L. (1994) *The Social Context of Health and Health Work*, London: Macmillan.

Klein, R. (1984) 'The Politics of Participation', in R. Maxwell and N. Weaver, *Public Participation in Health*, London: King's Fund.

Lalonde, M. (1974) *A New Perspective on the Health of Canadians*, Ottawa: Information Canada.

Larkin, G. (1995) 'State Control and the Health Professions in the United Kingdom: Historical Perspectives', in T. Johnson, G. Larkin and M. Saks (eds), *Health Professions and the State in Europe*, London: Routledge.

Lemmp, H. (1996) 'Class Act?', *Health Service Journal* 106 (5532): 30–31.

Light, D. (1995) 'Countervailing Powers: a Framework for Professions in Transition', cited in J. Loewenberg (1996) 'Industrial Relations Effects of English Health Care Reforms on Doctors', *International Journal of Health Services* 26 (4): 611–623.

Lowenberg, J. (1995) 'Health Promotion and the "Ideology of Choice"', *Public Health Nursing* 12 (5): 319–323.

—— (1996) 'Industrial Relations Effects of English Healthcare Reforms on Doctors', *International Journal of Health Services* 26 (4): 611–623.

McCormick, A., Charlton, J. and Fleming, D. (1995) 'Who Sees their General Practitioner and for What Reason?' *Health Trends* 27 (2): 34–35.

MacKenzie, W.J.M. (1979) *Power and Responsibility in Health Care*, Oxford: Oxford University Press.

McKeown, T. (1979) *The Role of Medicine: Dream, Mirage or Nemesis?*, Oxford: Blackwell.

Mackintosh, N. (1995) 'Self-empowerment in Health Promotion: a Realistic Target?', *British Journal of Nursing* 4 (21): 1273–1278.

Miles, A. (1991) *Women, Health and Medicine*, Milton Keynes: Open University Press.

Millar, B. (1996) 'On Goes the Muzzle', *Health Service Journal* 106 (5531): 11.

Moran, G. (1986) 'Radical Health Promotion: a Role for Local Authorities?', in S. Rodmell and A. Watt (eds), *The Politics of Health Education: Raising the Issues*, London: Routledge.
—— (1991) 'Fourth Time Around: NHS Reorganisation and Public Health', in P. Draper, *Health through Public Policy*, London: Green Print.
Moran, G. and Watkins, S. (1991) 'The Medical Guardians', in P. Draper, *Health through Public Policy*, London: Green Print.
NAHAT (1995/6) *NAHAT Handbook*,10th edn, Kent: JMH Publishing.
Naidoo, J. and Wills, J. (1994) *Health Promotion Foundations for Practice*, London: Bailliere Tindall.
Navarro, V. (1976) *Medicine under Capitalism*, New York: Prodist.
—— (1986) *Crisis, Health and Medicine: A Social Critique*, London: Tavistock.
Oakley, A. (1984) *The Captured Womb: A History of the Medical Care of Pregnant Women*, Oxford: Blackwell.
Richman, J. (1987) *Medicine and Health,* London: Longman
Rodmell, S. and Watt, A. (eds) (1986) *The Politics of Health Education: Raising the Issues*, London: Routledge.
Savage, W. (1986) *A Savage Enquiry: Who Controls Childbirth?*, London: Heinemann.
Townsend, P. and Davidson, N. (eds) (1982) *Inequalities in Health: The Black Report*, Harmondsworth: Penguin, repr. 1992.
Walt, G. (1994) *Health Policy: an Introduction to Process and Power*, London: Zed.
Whitehead, M. (1992) 'The Health Divide', in *Inequalities in Health*, Harmondsworth: Penguin.
Yen, L. (1995) 'From Alma Alta to Asda and Beyond: a Commentary on the Transition in Health Promotion Services in Primary Care from Commodity to Control', in R. Bunton, S. Nettleton and R. Burrows, *The Sociology of Health Promotion*, London: Routledge.
Zola, I. (1975) 'Medicine as an Institution of Social Control' in C. Cox and A. Mead (eds), *A Sociology of Medical Practice*, Gateshead: Collier-Macmillan.

Chapter 6

Bennett, P. and Murphy, S. (1994) 'Psychology and Health Promotion', *The Psychologist: Bulletin of the British Psychological Society* March: 126–130.
Benzeval, M., Judge, K. and Whitehead, M. (eds) (1995) *Tackling Inequalities in Health*, London: King's Fund.
Butler, J. (1993) *Evaluating the NHS Reforms*, London: King's Fund.
DOH (1992) *The Health of the Nation: A Strategy for Health in England*, London: HMSO.
Durkheim, É. (1870) *Suicide: A Study in Sociology*, ed. G. Simpson, London: Routledge & Kegan Paul, 1952.
Ewles, L. (1993) 'Hope Against Hype', *Health Service Journal* 103 (5367): 30.
Garbay, J. (1992) 'The Health of the Nation: Seize the Opportunity', *British Medical Journal* 305: 129–130.
Gray, M. (1991) 'In Poverty and in Health', *Health Service Journal* July: 24.
Grimley Evans, J. (1991) 'The Health of the Nation Responses: The Challenge of Ageing', *British Medical Journal* 303, August: 408.

Ham, C. (1993) *Health Policy in Britain*, 3rd edn, London: Macmillan.

Hawton, K. (1986) *Suicide and Attempted Suicide*, London: Sage.

—— (1993) 'By Their Own Young Hand', *British Medical Journal* 304: 1000.

Howarth, P.J.N. (1991) 'The Health of the Nation', *British Medical Journal* 308: 184.

Mckeown, K. (1995) '"Black to Basics": A Health Promotion Interpretation', *Society of Health Education and Health Promotion Specialists* 1 (1): 13–16.

Marmot, M.G. (1986) 'Mortality Decline and Widening Social Inequalities', *The Lancet* 2: 274–276.

Nocon, A. (1993) 'Health Alliances', *Health Service Journal* December: 24–28.

Parish, R. (1991) 'Policy or Public Procrastination: Part ii, The Implications for Health of the Nation', *Health Education Journal* 50 (3): 141–145.

Pearson, C. (1992) 'Missing Target', *Social Work Today* 23, August: 10.

Phillimore, P., Beattie, A. and Townsend, P. (1994) 'Widening Inequalities in Health in Northern England, 1981–1991', *British Medical Journal* 308: 1125–1128.

Platt, S. (1989) 'Depression and Suicide', *Health Service Journal* October: 36–40.

Platt, S. and Salter, D. (1990) 'Suicidal Intent, Hopelessness and Depression in a Parasuicide Population: the Influence of Social Desirability and Elapsed Time', *British Journal of Clinical Psychology* 29: 361–371.

Radical Statistics Health Group (1991a) 'Missing: a Strategy for Health of the Nation', *British Medical Journal* 303, August: 299–302.

—— (1991b) 'Let Them Eat Soap', *Health Service Journal* November: 25–28.

Robinson, R. (ed.) (1993) 'Evaluating the NHS Reforms Policy Journals', *Health Service Journal* 103 (5370): 27.

Savage, W. (1989) 'Women's Knowledge and Experience of Cervical Screening: A Failure of Health Education and Medical Organisation', *Community Medicine* 11 (4): 279–289.

Sheldon, T. (1990) 'When it Makes Sense To Mince Your Words', *Health Service Journal* 100: 1211.

Smith, R. (1991) 'The Health of the Nation Responses: First Step Towards a Strategy for Health', *British Medical Journal* 303: 297–298.

Townsend, P. and Davidson, N. (eds) (1982) *Inequalities in Health: The Black Report*, Harmondsworth: Penguin, repr. 1992.

Tudor Hart, J. (1971) 'The Inverse Care Law', *Lancet* i: 405.

Whitehead, M. (1982) 'The Health Divide', in P. Townsend, N. Davidson (eds) *Inequalities in Health*, Harmondsworth: Penguin.

Wilkinson, M.J. (1995) 'Love is Not A Marketable Commodity: New Public Health Management in the British NHS', *Journal of Advanced Nursing* 21: 980–987.

Wilkinson, R.G. (1986) *Socio-economic Differences in Mortality: Interpreting the Data and their Size and Trends. Class and Health: Research and Longitudinal Data*, London: Tavistock.

WHO (1978) *Primary Healthcare: Report of the International Conference on Primary Healthcare at Alma Ata, USSR, September 6–12*, Geneva: WHO Europe.

—— (1981) *Global Strategy for Health for All by the Year 2000*, Geneva: WHO Europe.

—— (1982) *Health Promotion: Concepts and Principles*, Geneva WHO.

—— (1984) 'Health Promotion: a Discussion Document on the Concepts and Principles', Copenhagen: WHO; repr. (1985) in *Journal of the Institute of Health Education* 23 (1).

—— (1986) *Ottawa Charter for Health Promotion*, Geneva: WHO.

—— (1992) *Health Promotion in Action*, Geneva: WHO.

Chapter 7

Adler, M. (1995) *ABC of Sexually Transmitted Diseases*, 3rd edn, London: British Medical Journal.

Aggleton, P. and Moody, D. (1992) 'Monitoring and Evaluation HIV/AIDS Health Education and Health Promotion', in P. Aggleton, *Does it Work* London: Health Education Authority.

Aggleton, P. and Tyrer P. (1994) *Sexual Health*, in P. Aggleton *et al.*, *Learning about AIDS*, ch. 5, 2nd edn, London: Churchill Livingstone.

Alcorn, K. (ed.) (1996) *AIDS Reference Manual*, London: NAM Publications.

Bloor, M. (1995) 'A User's Guide to Contrasting Theories of HIV Related Risk Behaviour', in J. Gabe, *Medicine, Health and Risk: Sociological Approaches*, Oxford: Blackwell.

Cohen, M. and Chwalow, J. (1995) 'The Health Belief Model: Always, Sometimes or Never Useful in Guiding HIV/AIDS Prevention', in D. Friedrich and W. Heckmann (ed.), *Aids in Europe: The Behavioural Aspect*, vol. 4, *Determinants of Behaviour Change*, Germany: Rosch-Buch, Hallstadt.

DOH (1992) *The Health of the Nation: A Strategy for Health in England*, London: HMSO.

Friedrich, L., Knox, M., Boaz, T. and Dow, M. (1994) 'HIV Risk Factors for Persons with Serious Mental Illness', *Community Mental Health Journal* 30 (6): 551–563.

Godfrey, C. and Tolley, K. (1992) 'An Economic Approach to the Evaluation of HIV/AIDS Health Education Programmes', in P. Aggleton, *Does it Work*, London: Health Education Authority.

Holland, J. and Fullerton, D. (1995) 'Establishing the Effectiveness of Behavioural Interventions to Prevent HIV: Some Trials and Tribulations', in D. Friedrich and W. Heckmann (ed.), *AIDS in Europe: The Behavioural Aspect*, vol. 4, *Determinants of Behaviour Change*, Germany: Rosch-Buch, Hallstadt.

Holland, J., Ramazanoglu, C., Scott, S., Sharpe, S. and Thomson, R. (1992) 'Pressure, Resistance, Empowerment: Young Women and the Negotiation of Safer Sex', in P. Aggleton, P. Davies and G. Hart, *AIDS: Rights, Risk and Reason*, London: Falmer Press.

Johnson, A. (1991) *HIV/AIDS in The Health of the Nation*, London: British Medical Journal.

Johnson, A., Wadsworth, J., Wellings, K. and Field, J. (1994) *The National Survey of Sexual Attitudes and Lifestyles*, Oxford: Blackwell Scientific.

Kickbusch, I. (1994) 'Introduction: Tell Me a Story', in A. Pederson, M. O'Neill and I. Rootman (eds), *Health Promotion in Canada: Provincial, National and International Perspectives*, Toronto: W.B. Saunders.

McEwan, R. and Bhopal, R. (1991) *HIV/AIDS Health Promotion for Young People: A Review of Theory, Principles and Practice*, Paper 12, London: Health Education Authority.

McHaffie, H. (1993) 'Improving Awareness', *Nursing Times* May 5, 89 (18): 29–31.

Mann, S., Smith, T. and Barton, S. (1996) 'Pelvic Inflammatory Disease', *International Journal of STD and AIDS* 7: 315–321.

Pye, K. (1990) *AIDS Programmes: Evaluation of AIDS Health Promotion Programmes, Concepts and the Cambridge Study*, Paper 7, London: Health Education Authority.

Scott, S. (1992) 'Evaluation may Change Your Life, but it Won't Solve All Your Problems, in P. Aggleton, *Does it Work,* London: Health Education Authority.

Scott, S. and Freeman, R. (1995) 'Prevention as a Problem of Modernity: the Example of HIV/AIDS', in J. Gabe, *Medicine, Health and Risk : Sociological Approaches*, Oxford: Blackwell.

Smith, A. and Jacobson, B. (ed.) (1988) *The Nation's Health: A Strategy for the 1990's*, London: King's Fund.

Tones, B. (1981) 'Health Education: Prevention or Subversion?', *RSH* 3: 413–416.

Wellings, K., Field, J., Johnson, A.M., Wadsworth, J. and Bradshaw, S. (1994) *Sexual Behaviour in Britain*, Harmondsworth: Penguin.

WHO (1986) *Ottawa Charter for Health Promotion*, Geneva: WHO.

Chapter 8

Advertising Association (1984) *Finding Out . . . About Advertising*, London: Advertising Association.

Anderson, D. (1986) 'Healthy Eating: the Evidence', in D. Anderson (ed.), *A Diet of Reason: Sense and Nonsense in the Healthy Eating Debate*, London: Social Affairs Unit.

Ardell, D.B. (1977) *High Level Wellness: An Alternative to Doctors, Drugs and Disease*, Emmaus, PA: Rodale Press.

Arthur, C. (1996) 'After the Hype, the Scientists' Verdict: CJD to Kill Hundreds', *Independent* November 26: 1.

Blight, C.M. and Scanlan, S. (1986) 'Regulating Cakes and Ale: Agricultural Intervention and Health, in D. Anderson (ed.), *A Diet of Reason: Sense and Nonsense in the Healthy Eating Debate,* London: Social Affairs Unit.

Brierley, H., Goddard, P. and Wildbore, A. (1988) 'Yes, We Have No Bananas, but Plenty of Health Care Today', *Health Visitor* 61 (12): 369–370.

British Heart Foundation (1996) *So You Want to Lose Weight: a Guide to Losing Weight for Men*, London: British Heart Foundation.

Brown, D. (1996) 'Super-food Sales set to "Rocket"', *Daily Telegraph* December 5: 9.

Brown, J.L. and Pollitt, E. (1996) 'Malnutrition, Poverty and Intellectual Development', *Scientific American* 274 (2): 26–31.

Bull, N. (1995) 'Dietary Habits of 15 to 25-year-olds', *Human Nutrition Applied* 39A (Suppl.): 1–68.

Burke, D. (1994) 'Ethical Questions on your Plate', *Church Times* July; in C. Donnellan (ed.) (1996) *Biotechnology: Friend or Foe?*, Cambridge: Independence.

Campbell, A.V. (1990) 'Education or Indoctrination? The Issue of Autonomy in Health Education', in S. Doxiasis (ed.), *Ethics in Health Education*, Chichester: Wiley.

Cannon, G. (1987) *The Politics of Food*, London: Century Hutchinson.

Caraher, M. (1994) 'Health Promotion: Time for an Audit', *Nursing Standard* 8 (20): 32–35.

Catford, J. and Ford, S. (1984) 'On the State of the Public Ill Health: Premature Mortality in the United Kingdom and Europe', *British Medical Journal* 289, December (15): 1668–1670.

Catford, J. and Parish, R. (1989) '"Heartbeat Wales": New Horizons for Health Promotion in the Community – the Philosophy and Practice of "Heartbeat Wales"' in D. Seedhouse and A. Cribb (eds), *Changing Ideas in Healthcare*, Chichester: Wiley.

Clover, C. (1996) 'Gummer Outlaws Genetically-altered American Maize', *Daily Telegraph* December 5: 9.

Daily Mail (1996) 'Good Health: The Dirty Dozen', December 3: 38.

DOH (1992) *The Health of the Nation: A Strategy for Health in England*, London: HMSO.

Donnellan, C. (ed.) (1996a) *Biotechnology – Friend or Foe?*, vol. 12, Cambridge: Independence.

—— (ed.) (1996b) *Body Image*, vol. 24, Cambridge: Independence.

Downie, R. (1983) 'Is there a Right to be Unhealthy?', *Nursing Mirror* 156 (8): 30.

Doyal, L. (1994) 'Changing Medicine? Gender and the Politics of Health Care' in J. Gabe, D. Kelleher and G. Williams (eds), *Challenging Medicine*, London: Routledge.

Driver, C. (1984) 'How the Poor Eat', *New Society* November 22.

Drummond, J.C., Wilbraham, A. and Hollingsworth, D. (1957) *The Englishman's Food: Five Centuries of English Diet*, London: Jonathan Cape.

Eaton, L. (1994) 'Taking the Biscuit', *Health Visitor* June, 67 (6): 187–188.

Emmett, S. (1996) 'Bulimia Cases Treble in Just Five Years' in *Independent on Sunday* 356, December 1: 1.

Epp, J. (1986) *Achieving Health for All: A Framework for Health Promotion*, Ottawa: Health and Welfare, Canada.

Geary, J. (1996) 'Battle of the Bean Genes', *Time* October 28, 148 (18): 48–49.

George, M. (1993) 'Poverty, Diet and Health', *Nursing Standard* 7 (49): 21–23.

Haller, J. (1994) *What to Eat When you Don't Feel like Eating*, Hansport, Nova Scotia: Lancelot Press.

Health and Welfare, Canada (1992) *Using the Food Guide*, Ottawa: Health and Welfare, Canada

Health Education Authority (1989) *Diet, Nutrition and 'Healthy Eating' in Low Income Groups*, London: Health Education Authority.

—— (1994) *Introducing the National Food Guide: the Balance of Good Health*, pamphlet, London: Health Education Authority.

Health Visitor (1991) 'Editorial: The Heart of the Matter' 64 (7): 205.

Health Visitors' Association (1991) '"The Health of the Nation": The HVA responds', *Health Visitor* 64 (11): 365–367.

Helman, C. (1984) *Health, Culture and Illness*, Bristol: Wright.

Jackson, C. (1992) 'It's all at the Shopping Co-op', *Health Visitor* 65 (10), October: 372.

Kelleher, D. (1994) 'Self-help Groups and their Relationship to Medicine' in J. Gabe, D. Kelleher and G. Williams (eds), *Challenging Medicine*, London: Routledge.

Kemm, J. and Close, A. (1995) *Health Promotion: Theory and Practice*, Basingstoke: Macmillan.

Labonte, R. (1989) 'Community and Professional Empowerment', *Canadian Nurse* 85(3): 23–26, 28.

Lancet (1986) 'Britain Needs a Food and Health Policy: the Government Must Face its Duty', *Lancet*, Reviews, 2 (8501), August 23: 434–436.

Le Fanu, J. (1986) 'Diet and Disease: Nonsense and Nonscience', in D. Anderson (ed), *A Diet of Reason: Sense and Nonsense in the Healthy Eating Debate*, London: Social Affairs Unit.

Lobstein, T. (1991) 'Diet and Disease Revisited', *Health Visitor* 64 (6), June: 176.

—— (1993) 'Milking the Market', *Health Visitor* 66 (7), July: 266.

—— (1994) 'Pulling the Strings of World Food Trade', *Health Visitor* 67 (4): 143.

—— (1995) 'Something Fishy in the Milk Formula', *Health Visitor* 68 (3): 117.

Lupton, D. (1996) *Food, the Body and the Self*, London: Sage.

Lyman, B. (1989) *A Psychology of Food: More than a Matter of Taste*, New York: Van Nostrand Reinhold.

Mares, P., Henley, A. and Baxter, C. (1985) *Health Care in Multicultural Britain*, Cambridge: Health Education Council and the National Extension College.

Marks, V. (1991) *Is British Food Bad for You?*, London: IEA Health and Welfare Unit.

Naegele, B. (1992) 'Canada's Framework for Health Promotion and Chronic Illness', in *Health Promotion and Chronic Illness: Discovering a New Quality of Health*, Copenhagen: WHO Regional Office for Europe (in collaboration with the Federal Centre for Health Education, Cologne).

Open University (1985) *The Open University Guide to Healthy Eating*, London: Rambletree Pelham (in association with The Health Education Council and the Scottish Health Education Group).

Pearce, F. (1996) 'Greedy Patenting could Starve Poor of Biotech Promise', *New Scientist* 152 (2056) November 16: 6.

Potrykus, C. (1989) 'HEA Refuses to Publish Report Linking Unhealthy Diet to Poverty', *Health Visitor* 62 (12): 359.

—— (1991) 'Soft Sell for Hard-pressed Teachers', *Health Visitor* 64 (5): 138.

Robbins, C. (1991) 'Our Manufactured Diet', in P. Draper (ed.), *Health Through Public Policy: The Greening of Public Health*, London: Greenprint.

Robin, N. (1991) 'The Heart of the Matter', Editorial, *Health Visitor* 64 (7): 205.

Royal College of Nursing (1991) *The Health of the Nation: A Response from the Royal College of Nursing*, London: Ren.

Scott-Samuel, A. (ed.) (1990) *Total Participation: Total Health. Reinventing the Peckham Health Centre for the 1990s*, Guildford: Pioneer Health Centre.

Smith, A. and Jacobson, B. (1988) *The Nations' Health. A Strategy for the 1990s*, London: King's Fund.

Smith, C. and Roberts, C. (1994) 'Health-related Behaviour in Wales, 1985–1990', *Health Trends* 26 (1): 18–21.

Spens, C. (1996) 'Health of the Nation: Promoting a Healthy Lifestyle', *Health Visitor* 69 (10), October: 429–430.

Taylor, J. and Taylor, D. (eds) (1990) *Safe Food Handbook*, London: Ebury Press.

Townsend, P. and Davidson, N. (eds) (1982) *Inequalities in Health: The Black Report*, Harmondsworth: Penguin, repr. 1992.

Usher, R. (1996) 'A Tall Story for our Time', *Time* 148 (16): 88–94.

Walker, C. and Cannon, G. (1985) *The Food Scandal*, London: Century.

West London Healthcare NHS Trust/West London Health Promotion Agency (1996) *Healthy Eating for Asian People*, pamphlet, London: West London Healthcare NHS Trust/West London Health Promotion Agency.

Which? (1995) 'Food poisoning', *Which?* September: 8–11.

—— (1996) 'BSE – Where Now?', *Which?* May: 58

WHO (1986) *Ottawa Charter for Health Promotion*, Geneva: WHO.

Chapter 9

Anderson, R., Jones, T. and Thorneycroft, C. (1991) 'Learning to Empower Patients', *Diabetes Care* 14: 585–590.

Beauchamp, T. and Childress, J. (1994) *Principles of Biomedical Ethics*, Oxford: Oxford University Press.

Blackburn, C. (1991) *Poverty and Health: Working With Families*, Milton Keynes: Open University Press.

Blaxter, M. (1990) *Health and Lifestyles*, London: Tavistock.

Campbell, A. (1993) 'The Ethics of Health Education', Ch. 3 in J. Wilson Barnett and J. Macleod Clark, *Research in Health Promotion and Nursing*, London: Macmillan.

Chadwick, R. and Tadd, W. (1992) *Ethics and Nursing Practice: A Case Study Approach*, London: Macmillan.

Conrad, P. (1985) 'The Meaning of Medications: Another Look at Compliance', *Social Science Medicine* 20 (1): 29–37.

Davies, B. (1991) *Community Health and Social Services* Sevenoaks: Edward Arnold.

DOH (1991) *The Patient's Charter*, London: HMSO.

Dougherty, C. (1993) 'Bad Faith and Victim-Blaming: The Limits of Health Promotion', *Health Care Analysis* 1: 111–119.

Douglas, J. (1960) '"Premature" Children at Primary Schools', *British Medical Journal* April/June: 1008–1013.

Egger, M., Brandt, F. and Muir, J. (1992) 'Human Insulin and Awareness of Hypoglycaemia: The Need for a Large Randomised Trial', *British Medical Journal* 305: 351–355.

Ellis, P. (1993) 'Role of Ethics in Modern Healthcare', *British Journal of Nursing* 2 (2): 144–146.

Faulder, C. (1985) *Whose Body is it?: The Troubling Issue of Informed Consent*, London: Virago.

Fitzpatrick, R. (1989) 'Lay Concepts of Illness', in P. Brown (ed.), *Perspectives in Medical Sociology*, Belmont, CA: Wadsworth.

Gillon, R. (1994) 'Medical Ethics: Four Principles plus Attention to Scope', *British Medical Journal* 309: 184–188.

Ginzberg, E. (1977) 'The Sacred Cows of Health Manpower', *Man and Medicine* 2: 235–242.

Grant, D. and Manyande, A. (1994) 'Care of People with Long-term Illness', in V. Tschudin (ed.), *Ethics: Nursing People with Special Needs*, London: Scutari Press.

Harris, J. (1985) *The Value of Life*, London: Routledge & Kegan Paul.

Hart, J. (1994) *Feasible Socialism*, London: Socialist Health Association.

Holden, R. (1990) 'Empathy: The Art of Emotional Knowing in Holistic Nursing Care', *Holistic Nurse Practice* 5: 70–79.

Holder, A. (1981) 'Informed Consent and the Nurse', *Nursing Law and Ethics* 2: 1–2, 8.

Holm, S. (1993) 'What is Wrong with Compliance?', *Journal of Medical Ethics* 19: 108–110.

Illich, I. (1976) *Limits to Medicine: Medical Nemesis – The Expropriation of Health*, London: Marion Boyars.

Kelleher, D. (1988) 'Coming to Terms with Diabetes: Coping Strategies and Non-compliance', in R. Anderson and M. Bury (eds), *Living with Chronic Illness: The Experience of Patients and their Families*, London: Unwin Hyman.

Kuhn, T. (1977) *The Essential Tension: Selected Studies in Scientific Tradition and Change*, Chicago, IL: University of Chicago Press.

MacDonald, T. (1994) 'Osteopathy as Health Promotion: A Semantic Analysis', *British Osteopathy Journal* 14: 30–32.

Mill, J.S. (1859) 'On Liberty' in *Three Essays*, Oxford: Oxford University Press, pp. 5–141, 1975.

Moore, K. (1995) 'Compliance or Collaboration? The Meaning for the Patient', *Nursing Ethics* 2: 71–76.

Morgan, M. (1991) 'The Doctor–Patient Relationship', G. Scambler (ed.), *Sociology as Applied to Medicine*, London: Bailliere Tindall, pp. 47–64.

Morse, J., Bottorf, J., Anderson, G., O'Brien, B. and Solberg, S. (1992) 'Beyond Empathy: Expanding Expressions of Caring', *Journal of Advanced Nursing* 17: 809–821.

O'Neill, O. (1984) 'Paternalism and Partial Autonomy in Medicine', *The Journal of Medical Ethics* 10: 173–178.

Parsons, T. (1951) *The Social System*, London: Routledge & Kegan Paul.

Pellegrino, E. (1979) 'Towards a Reconstruction of Medical Morality: The Primacy of the Act of Profession and the Fact of Illness', *Journal of Medicine and Philosophy* 4: 32–56.

Raven, B. (1988) 'Social Power and Compliance in Health Care', in S. Maes, C.D. Spielberger, P.B. Defares and I.G. Sarason (eds), *Topics of Health Psychology*, London: Wiley.

Rowson, R. (1990) *An Introduction to Ethics for Nurses*, London: Scutari Press.

Ryan, T. (1994) 'Interpretations of Illness and Non-compliance with Nursing Care', *British Journal of Nursing* 3 (4): 163–167.

Seedhouse, D. (1988) *Ethics: The Heart of Health Care*, London: Wiley.

Shillitoe, R. (1995) 'Diabetes Mellitus', in A. Broome and S. Llewelyn (eds), *Health Psychology: Processes and Applications*, London: Chapman & Hall.

Strong, P. (1979) *The Ceremonial Order of the Clinic*, London: Routledge & Kegan Paul.

Tattersall, R. (1992) 'Human Insulin Gone Wrong', *Diabetes Medicine* 9: 397.

Trostle, A. (1989) 'Beneficence and the Social Worker', *Social Work in Health Care* 14 (2): 81–98.

Waitzkin, H. (1989) 'A Critical Theory of Medical Discourse: Ideology, Social Control, and the Processing of Social Context in Medical Encounters', *Journal of Social Behaviour* 30: 220–239.

Williams, G. and Wood, P. (1986) 'Commonsense Beliefs about Illness: A Mediating Role for the Doctor', *Lancet* 2: 1435–1437.

WHO (1986) *Ottawa Charter for Health Promotion*, Geneva: WHO.

Yeo, M. (1993) 'Toward an Ethic of Empowerment for Health Promotion', *Health Promotion International* 8 (3): 225–235.

Chapter 10

Aitken, S. (1985) 'Deconstructing the Media', in *Anthology of Literary Criticism*, New York: Ultima, pp.175–198.

Berridge, V. (1991) 'Aids, the Media and Health Policy', *Health Education Journal* 50 (4): 179–186.

Brown, W. and Basil, M. (1995) 'Media Celebrities and Public Health: Response to "Magic" Johnson's HIV Disclosure and its Impact on AIDS Risk and High Risk Behaviours', *Health Communication* 7 (4): 345–370.

Dignan, M., Bahnson, J., Sharpe, P., Beal, P., Smith, M. and Michielutte, R. (1991) 'Implementation of Mass Media Community Health Education: the Forsyth County Cervical Cancer Prevention Project', *Health Education Research* 6 (3): 259–266.

Egger, M. and Timsett, N. (1993) *Health and the Media: Principles and Practices for Health Promotion*, Sydney: McGraw Hill.

Farquhar, J. and Fortman, S. (1984) 'Effects of Community-wide Education on Cardiovascular Disease Risk Factors', *Journal of the American Medical Association* 264: 359–365.

Flora, J. and Wallack, L. (1990) 'Health Promotion and the Mass Media Use: Translating Research into Practice', *Health Education Research* 5 (1): 73–80.

Freedman, S. (1984) 'Much Ado About Headaches', *School Health Magazine* 41 (Winter): 75–81.

Froberg, D., Williams, C. and Mate, N. (1986) 'Project Mental Health: a Case Study of a Mass Media Health Promotion Program', *Health Education Research* 1 (4): 315–323.

Hastings, G. and Haywood, A. (1991) 'Social Marketing and Communication in Health Promotion', *Health Promotion International* 6 (2): 135–145.

Katz, A. and Lazarsfield, D. (1995) 'Epidemics and the Media', *American Journal of Media Studies* 16 (5): 19–26.

Klaidman, S. (1990) *How Well the Media Report Health Risk*, New York: Daedalus.

Klapper, T. (1961) *When News Doesn't Fit*, vol. 3, *Studies of the Hearst Press*, Wheeling VA: Rasper Bookhouse.

Maccoby, C. and Fenner, T. (1977) 'Use of Media for Health Education in Three California Cities', in *We, the People*, Stanford, CA: Stanford University Press.

Maccoby, E. (1980) *Social Development*, New York: Harcourt Brace Jovanovich.

McGuire, J. (1986a) 'Impact of Newspaper Reporting on Health Beliefs', in *Role of the Media in Modern Society*, Mountain View, CA: Mayfield.

—— (1986b) 'Press report on the AIDS Scare', *World Health Forum* 7: 42–45.

Molitor, F. (1993) 'Accuracy in Science News Reporting by Newspapers: The Case of Aspirin for the Prevention of Heart Attacks', *Health Communication* 5 (3): 209–224.

New England Journal of Medicine (1988) 'Editorial: What Price Accuracy', 310: 1.

New York Daily News (1988) 'New Breakthrough in Heart Health', 6 August: 4.

Pierce, R. and Daveluy, C. (1986) *La Planification de la santé*, Montreal: Agence d'arc.

Puska, R. and Dornbush, S. (1985) 'Segmenting Estimates of Health Risk in Finland', *Health Promotion International* 9 (4): 289–296.

Redman, S., Spencer, E. and Sanson-Fisher, W. (1990) 'The Role of the Mass Media in Changing Health-related Behaviour: a Critical Appraisal of Two Models', *Health Promotion International* 5 (1): 85–103.

Relman, A. (1988) 'Aspirin for the Primary Prevention of Myocardial Infarction', *The New England Journal of Medicine* 318: 245–246.

Roberts, W. and Maccoby, N. (1985) 'Community Education for Healthy Living: A Project Design', *American Journal of Epidemiology* 122: 323–334.

Rose, G. (1993) *The Strategy of Preventive Medicine*, New York: Oxford University Press.

Shelley, J., Irwig, L., Simpson, J. and Macaskill, P. (1991) 'Evaluation of a Mass-media-led Campaign to Increase Pap Smear Screening', *Health Education Research* 6 (3): 267–277.

Sorlin, M. (1994) 'Duties in Health Reporting', *Journal of Applied Psychology* 78 (6), October: 763–773.

Tones, K. (1990) 'Positive Health', *Nursing* 4 (22): 33–35.

Wallack, L. (1990) 'Two Approaches to Health Promotion in the Mass Media', *World Health Forum* 11: 143–154.

Wallack, L., Dorfman, L., Jernigan, D. and Themba, M. (1993) *Media Advocacy and Public Health Power for Prevention*, London: Sage.

Chapter 11

Ashton, D. (1989) *The Corporate Healthcare Revolution*, London: Kogan Page.

Ashton, I. and Gill, F. (1991) *Monitoring for Health Hazards at Work*, 2nd edn, Oxford: Blackwell.

Astor, J.J. (1972) *The Third Winter of Unemployment*, cited in Constantine (1980) *Unemployment Between Wars*.

Bartley, M. (1994) 'Unemployment and Ill Health: Understanding the Relationship' *Journal of Epidemiology and Community Health* 48: 333–337.

Baum, A., Fleming, R. and Reddy, D.M. (1986) 'Unemployment Stress: Loss of Control, Reactance and Learned Helplessness', *Social Science and Medicine* 22 (5): 509–516.

Beale, V. and Nethercott, C. (1987) 'The Health of Industrial Employees Four Years after Compulsory Redundancy', *Journal of the Royal College of General Practitioners* 37: 390–394.

—— (1988) 'The Nature of Unemployment Morbidity', *Journal of the Royal College of General Practitioners*, 38: 200–202.

Beer, M. (1990) 'Why Change Programmes Don't Produce Change', *Harvard Business Review* November/December: 214–222.

Benzeval, M., Judge, K. and Whitehead, M. (1995) *Tackling Inequalities in Health*, London: King's Fund.

Bertera, R. (1991) 'Planning and Implementing Health Promotion in the Workplace: A Case Study of the Du Pont Company Experience', *Health Education Quarterly* 17, Fall (3): 307–327.

Best, R. (1995) 'The Housing Dimension', in M. Benzeval, K. Judge and M. Whitehead (eds), *Tackling Inequalities in Health: An Agenda for Action*, London: King's Fund.

Blackburn, C. (1991) *Poverty and Health: Working With Families*, Milton Keynes: Open University Press.

Blaxter, M. (1990) *Health and Lifestyles*, London: Routledge.

Bovell, V. (1992) 'The Economic Benefits of Health Promotion in the Workplace', in *Action on Health at Work Seminar, 18th February*, London: Health Education Authority.

Burchell, B. (1994) 'The Effects of Labour Market Position, Job Insecurity, and Unemployment on Psychological Health', in D. Gallie, C. March and C. Vogler (eds), *Social Change and the Experience of Unemployment*, Oxford: Oxford University Press.

Canton, J. (1984) *Health Promotion in the Workplace*, eds M. O'Donnell and T. Ainsworth, Chicago, IL: Wiley Medical Publication.

Clark, A. and Layard, R. (1993) *UK Unemployment*, 2nd edn, Oxford: Heinemann.

Conrad, P. (1988) 'Worksite Health Promotion: The Social Context', *Social Science and Medicine* 26 (5): 485–489.

Constantine, S. (1980) *Unemployment Between the Wars*, Harlow: Longman.

Convery, P. (1996) '60% of Claimant Count Fall is "Administrative" says Government', *Working Brief* December 1996/January 1997: 25–28.

Cooper, S. (1995) 'Unemployment and Health', *British Journal of Nursing* 4: 566–569.

Dedman, R. (1986) *Kimberly Clark Health Management Programme in Health Care Cost Containment*, eds A. Conway and C. Leibman, Philadelphia, PA: Leonard Davies Institute of Health Economics.

DOH (1992) *The Health of the Nation: A Strategy for Health in England*, London: HMSO.

Drucker, P. (1969) *The Age of Discontinuity*, London: Heinemann.

Duck, J. (1993) 'Managing Change: The Art of Balancing', *Harvard Business Review* November/December: 95–101.

Dyer, W. (1984) *Strategies for Managing Change*, Boston, MA: Addison-Wesley.

Fagin, L. and Little, M. (1984) *The Forsaken Families: The Effects of Unemployment on Family Life*, London: Penguin.

Farquhar, J. (1978) *The American Way of Life Need Not Be Hazardous to Your Health*, New York: Norton.

Fox, A. and Adelstein, A. (1978) 'Occupational Mortality: Work or a Way of Life?', *Journal of Epidemiology and Community Health* 33: 73–78.

Friedlander, F. (1975) 'Emergent and Contemporary Life Styles: An Intergenerational Issue', *Human Relations* 28 (4): 329–347.

Fukuyama, F. (1992) *The End of History and the Last Man*, London: Hamish Hamilton.

Gallie, D. and Vogler, C. (1994) 'Unemployment and Attitudes to Work', in D. Gallie, C. Marsh and C. Vogler (eds) *Social Change and the Experience of Unemployment*, Oxford: Oxford University Press.

Gallie, D., Marsh, C. and Vogler, C. (eds) (1994) *Social Change and the Experience of Unemployment*, Oxford: Oxford University Press.

Gershuny, J. (1994) 'The Psychological Consequences of Unemployment: An Assessment of the Jahoda Thesis', in D. Gallie, C. Marsh and C. Vogler (eds) *Social Change and the Experience of Unemployment*, Oxford: Oxford University Press.

Gershuny, J. and Marsh, C. (1994) 'Unemployment in Work Histories', in D. Gallie, C. Marsh and C. Vogler (eds) *Social Change and the Experience of Unemployment*, Oxford: Oxford University Press.

Hammond, J. and Hammond, B. (1910) *The Town Labourer*, London: Macmillan.

Hammond, J. and Hammond, B. (1910) *The Village Labourer*, London: Macmillan.

Harvey, S. (1988) *Just an Occupational Hazard? Policies for Health at Work*, London: King's Fund.

Health Education Authority (1993) *Health Promotion in the Workplace: A Summary*, London: Health Education Authority.

Hollander, R. and Lagerman, M. (1988) 'Corporate Characteristics and Worksite Health Promotion Programmes: Fortune 500 Survey Findings', *Social Science and Medicine* 26: 491.

Jacobson, B., Babb, P., Schilling, R. and Webb, T. (1988) *Health at Work? A Report on Health Promotion at the Workplace*, Research Report No. 22, London: Health Education Authority.

Jacobson, B., Smith, A. and Whitehead, M. (1991) *The Nation's Health: A Strategy for the 1990s*, London: King's Fund.

Jahoda, M. (1982) *Employment and Unemployment: A Social-Psychological Analysis*, Cambridge: Cambridge University Press.

Johnson, R. (1986) 'Holistic Lifestyles and Gender', *Contemporary Issues* 5 (April).

Layard, R., Nickell, S. and Jackman, R. (1994) *The Unemployment Crisis*, Oxford: Oxford University Press.

Lee, A.J., Crombie, I.K., Smith, W.C.S. and Tunstall-Pedhoe, H.D. (1991) 'Cigarette Smoking and Employment Status', *Social Science and Medicine* 32: 1309–1312.

Lisle, J. (1993) 'Independent Multidisciplinary Committee', in B. Jacobson, A. Smith and M. Whitehead (eds), *The Nation's Health: A Strategy for the 1990s*, London: King's Fund.

Ministry of Health (1929) *Investigation in the Coalfields of South Wales*, Cmd 3272; in S. Constantine, *Unemployment Between the Wars*, Harlow: Longman, 1980.

Morris, J., Cook, D. and Shaper, A. (1992) 'Non-employment and Changes in Smoking, Drinking and Body Weight', *British Medical Journal* 304: 536–541.

—— (1994) 'Loss of Employment and Mortality', *British Medical Journal* 308: 1135–1139.

Moser, K., Goldblatt, P., Fox, J. and Jones, D. (1987) 'Unemployment and Mortality: Comparison of the 1971 and 1981 Longitudinal Study Census Samples', *British Medical Journal* 294: 86–90.

Moser, K., Goldblatt, P. and Jones, D. (1990) 'Unemployment and Mortality', in P. Goldblatt (ed.), *Longitudinal Study 1971–1981: Mortality and Social Organisation*, London: HMSO, pp. 82–96.

Naidoo, J. and Wills, J. (1994) *Health Promotion: Foundations for Practice*, London: Bailliere Tindall.

Nelson-Jones, R. (1994) *The Theory and Practice of Counselling Psychology*, New York: Cassell Education.

Nettleton, S. (1995) *The Sociology of Health and Illness*, Oxford: Blackwell.

Nimmo, M. (1996) 'Welfare Myths Challenged by Government's own Research', *Working Brief* December 1996/January 1997: 19–22.

Owen, A.D.K. (1932) *A Report on Unemployment in Sheffield* Sheffield: Sheffield Social Survey Committee; in S. Constantine, *Unemployment Between the Wars*, Harlow: Longman, 1980.

Penack, M. (1991) 'Workplace Health Promotion Programmes: An Overview', *Nursing Clinics of North America* 26 (1): 233–240.

Philo, S. and Freedman, S. (1992) *Health at Work: A Needs Assessment in South West Thames Regional Health Authority*, London: SWTRHA.

Rajecki, D. (1990) 'Attitudes – Themes and Advances', in D. Bernstein, E. Roy, T. Strull and C. Wickens (eds), *Psychology*, Boston, MA: Houghton-Mifflin Company, 1991.

Sanders, D. (1993) *Workplace Health Promotion: A Review of the Literature. Directorate of Health Policy and Public Health*, Oxford: Regional Health Authority.

Smith, R. (1987) *Unemployment and Health: A Disaster and a Challenge*, Oxford: Oxford University Press.

Stoute, H. (1989) 'Can Health Screening Damage your Health?', *Journal of the Royal College of General Practitioners*, 39: 193–195.

Taylor, P. (1974) 'Sickness Absence: Facts and Misconceptions', *Journal of the Royal College of Physicians* 8 (4): 315–333.

Tones, K. (1990) *Health Education: Effectiveness and Efficiency*, London: Chapman & Hall.

Townsend, T. and Davidson, N. (eds) (1982) *Inequalities in Health: The Black Report*, Harmondsworth: Penguin, repr. 1992

Unemployment and Health Study Group (1984) *Unemployment, Health and Social Policy*, Leeds: Nuffield Centre for Health Services Studies, The University of Leeds.

US Department of Health and Human Services (1985) *The Health Consequences of Smoking: Chronic Obstructive Lung Disease*, London: Office on Smoking and Health, DHSS Publication No 84–50205.

Vagero, D. (1991) 'Inequality in Health: Some Theoretical and Empirical Problems', *Social Science and Medicine* 32 (4): 367–371.

Warr, P. (1985) 'Twelve Questions About Unemployment and Health', in B. Roberts, R. Finnegan and D. Gallie (eds), *New Approaches to Economic Life*, Manchester: Manchester University Press.

Warr, P. and Jackson, T. (1985) 'Factors Influencing the Psychological Impact of Unemployment and of Re-employment', *Psychological Medicine* 15; 795–807.

Watson, N. (1992) *Provision of Employee Health and Welfare Programmes in Public and Private Sector Organisations in the UK*, Sunderland: University of Sunderland.

West, P. and Sweeting, H. (1996) 'Nae Job, Nae Future: Young People and Health in a Context of Unemployment', *Health and Social Care in the Community* 4 (1): 50–62.

WHO (1984) 'Health Promotion: a WHO Discussion Document on the Concept and Principles'; repr. in *Journal of the Institute of Health Education* 23 (1): 5–9, 1985.

Wilson, S.H. and Walker, G.M. (1993) 'Unemployment and Health: A Review', *Public Health* 107: 153–162.

Chapter 12

Ahmed, M. and Hilton, T. (1982) 'How to Help Patients Stop Smoking', *American Family Physician* 25: 133–136.

Bandura, A. (1986) *Self-efficacy: in Social Foundations of Thought and Action*, Engelwood Cliffs, NJ: Prentice Hall.

Bradford, M. and Winn, S. (1993) 'A Survey of Practice Nurses' Views of Health Promotion', *Health Education Journal* 52 (2): 91–95

Brownell, K., Marlatt, G. and Lichenstein, E. (1986) 'Understanding and Preventing Relapse', *American Psychology* 41: 765–782.

Calnan, M. and Williams, S. (1993) 'Coronary Heart Disease Prevention: The Role of the General Practitioner', *Family Practice* 10 (2): 22–34.

Damrosch, S. (1991) 'General Strategies for Motivating People to Change their Behaviour', *Nursing Clinics of North America* 26 (4): 833–843.

DHSS (1987) *Promoting Better Health: The Government's Programme for Improving Primary Health Care*, London: HMSO.

—— (1989) *Working For Patients*, London: HMSO.

—— (1993) *Prevention and Health: Everyone's Business*, London: HMSO.

DiNicola, N. and DiMatteo, M. (1984) 'Practitioners, Patient and Compliance with Medical Regimens: A Social Psychological Perspective', in A. Baun, *Social Psychological Aspects of Health*, Hillsdale, NJ: Cooper Books.

Dobbs, J. and Marsh, A. (1983) *Smoking among Secondary School Children*, London: HMSO.

DOH (1990) 'Statistics for General Medical Practitioners in England and Wales – 1978–1988', *Statistical Bulletin* 4: 9.

—— (1992) *The Health of the Nation: A Strategy for Health in England*, London: HMSO.

—— (1993a) *Better Living, Better Life*, London: HMSO.

—— (1993b) *NHS Management Executive: Guidance for GP Contract Health Promotion Package*, London: HMSO.

Doll, R. and Hill, A. (1958) 'Smoking and Carcinoma of the Lung: Preliminary Report', *British Medical Journal* 2: 1271–1286.

—— (1964) 'Mortality in Relation to Smoking: Ten Years Observation of British Doctors', *British Medical Journal* 1: 1399–1410 and 1460–1467.

Family Heart Study Group (1994) 'Randomised Controlled Trial Evaluating Cardiovascular Screening and Intervention in General Practice: Principal Results of British Family Heart Study', *British Medical Journal* 308: 313–320.

Fowler, G. (1993) 'Educating Doctors in Smoking Cessation', *Tobacco Control* 2 (1): 5–6.

Fry, J. (1991) 'The New Contract: Is It Working?', *Update* July 15: 71–75.

Fullard, E., Fowler, G. and Gray, M. (1984) 'Facilitating Prevention in Primary Care', *British Medical Journal* 297: 1585–1587.

—— (1987) 'Promoting Prevention in Primary Care: Controlled Trial of Low Technology, Low Cost Approach', *British Medical Journal* 294: 1080–1082.

Gilpen, J., Pierce, J. and Burns, D. (1992) 'Trends in Physicians Giving Advice to Stop Smoking, US 1974–87', *Tobacco Control* 1: 31–36.

Gott, M. (1990) 'Policy Framework for Health Promotion', *Nursing Standard* September, 26: 5.

Gott, M. and O'Brian, P. (1990) 'The Role of the Nurse in Health Promotion', *Health Promotion International* 5 (2): 137–143.

Heather, N. (1989) 'Psychology and Brief Interventions', *British Journal of Addiction* 84 (4): 357–370.

Hughes, D. (1993) 'General Practitioners and the New Contract: Promoting Better Health through Financial Incentives', *Health Policy* 25: 39–50.

Hughes, D. and Yule, B. (1993) 'The Effect of Per-item Payments on the Behaviour of the General Practitioners', *Journal of the Royal College of General Practitioners* 36: 517–521.

International Agency for Research on Cancer (1986) *Tobacco Smoking*, Lyon: IARC.

James, R. and Herbert, S. (1992) 'Patient Characteristics and the Effect of Three Physician Delivered Smoking Interventions, *Preventive Medicine* 21: 557–573.

Jamrozik, K., Vessey, M., Fowler, G. and Van-Vunakis, H. (1984) 'Controlled Trial of Three Different Anti-smoking Interventions in General Practice, *British Medical Journal* 288: 1499–1503.

Janis, I. and Feshbach, S. (1953) *Effects of Fear-arousing Communications*; cited in S. Damrosch, 'General Strategies for Motivating People to Change their Behaviour', *Nursing Clinics of North America* 26: 4, 1991.

Janz, N. and Becker, M. (1984) 'The Health Belief Model: A Decade Later', *Health Education Quarterly* 11: 1–47.

Job, R. (1988) 'Effective and Ineffective Use of Fear in Health Promotion Campaigns', *American Journal of Public Health* 78: 163–167.

Kottke, T. (1988) 'Attributes of Successful Smoking Interventions in Medical Practice: A Meta-analysis of 39 Controlled Trials', *Journal of the American Medical Association* 259 (19): 2883–2889.

Lennox, A. (1992) 'Determinants of Outcome in Smoking Cessation', *British Journal of General Practice* 42: 247–252.

Lichtenstein, E., Ransom, C. and Brown, R. (1981) 'Effects of Counsellor Smoking Status on the Credibility of Smoking Cessation Programmes', *Journal of Drug Education* 11: 361–367.

Macleod Clark, J., Haverty, S., Eliot, K. and Kendall, S. (1985) *Helping People to Stop Smoking: The Nurse's Role*, London: Department of Nursing Studies, King's College, University of London.

Macleod Clark, J., Kendall, S. and Haverty, S. (1987) 'Effective Use of Health Education Skills', *The Professional Nurse* February: 136–139.

Ockene, J. (1987) 'Physician Delivered Interventions for Smoking Cessation: Strategies for Increasing Effectiveness', *Preventive Medicine* 16 (5): 723–737.

OPCS (1990) *Cigarette Smoking 1972–1988*, OPCS Monitor SS 90/7, London: OPCS.

OXCHECK: Imperial Cancer Research Fund Study Group (1994) 'Effectiveness of Health Checks Done by Nurses in Primary Care', *British Medical Journal* 308: 308–312.

Prochaska, J. and DiClemente, C. (1984) 'Stages and Processes of Self-change in Smoking: Towards an Integrative Model of Change', *Journal of Clinical Psychology* 51: 390–395.

Richmond, R. and Webster, I. (1985) 'A Smoking Cessation Programme for use in General Practices', *Medical Journal of Australia* 142: 190–194.

—— (1990) 'Can Your GP Help you Give up Smoking?', *Healthy Australia* 2 (3): 103–105

Richmond, R., Austin, A. and Webster, I. (1988) 'Three Year Evaluation of a Programme by General Practitioners to Help Patients to Stop Smoking', *British Medical Journal* 252: 803–806.

Ross, F., Bower, P. and Sibbald, B. (1994) 'Practice Nurses: Characteristics, Workload and Training Needs', *British Journal of General Practice* 44: 15–18.

Royal College of General Practitioners (1981) *Prevention of Arterial Disease in Practice*, GP no.19, London: Royal College of General Practitioners.

Royal College of Nursing (1984) *Training Needs of Practice Nurses*, London: RCN.

Russell, M. and Stapleton, J. (1983) 'Effect of Nicotine Gum as an Adjunct to General Practitioners' Advice Against Smoking', *British Medical Journal* 287: 1782–1785.

—— (1987) 'District Programme to Reduce Smoking', *Journal of Epidemiology and Community Health* 42: 111–115.

Russell, M., Stapleton, J., Jackson, P. and Belcher, M. (1988) 'District Programme to Reduce Smoking: Can Sustained Intervention by General Practitioners Affect Prevalence?', *Journal of Epidemiology and Community Health* 3: 111–115

Russell, M., Wilson, C., Taylor, C. and Baker, C. (1979) 'Effect of General Practitioners' Advice Against Smoking', *British Medical Journal* 2: 231–235.

Sanders, D. (1992) *Smoking Cessation Interventions: Is Patient Education Effective?*, London: Department of Public Health Policy.

Sanders, D., Fowler, G. and Mant, D.(1989) 'Randomised Controlled Trial of Anti-smoking Advice by Nurses in General Practice', *Journal of the Royal College of General Practitioners* 39: 273–276.

Shurtleff, S. (1974) 'Stratified Sampling for Risk Factors in the Framingham Cohorts', *American Statistical Bulletin* 7 (2): 391–398.

Slama, K. and Redman, S. (1990) 'The Effectiveness of Two Smoking Cessation Programmes for Use in General Practice', *British Medical Journal* 300: 1707–1709.

Stewart, P. and Rosser, W. (1982) 'The Impact of Routine Advice on Smoking Cessation from Family Physicians', *Canadian Medical Association Journal* 126: 1051–1054.

Stilwell, B. (1991) 'The Rise of the Practice Nurse', *Nursing Times* 87: 26–28.

Tudor Hart, J. (1971) 'The Inverse Care Law', *Lancet* i: 405.

Wald, N. and Nicolaides-Bouman, A. (eds) (1991) *UK Smoking Statistics*, Oxford: Oxford University Press.

Whitehead, M. (1987) *The Health Divide: Social Inequalities in Health*, London: HEA.

Chapter 13

Alcohol Alert No. 33 (1996) National Institute of Alcohol Abuse and Alcoholism, USA.

Alcohol Concern (1991) *Warning: Alcohol Can Damage Your Health*, London: Alcohol Concern.

American Psychiatric Association (1988) *Diagnostic and Statistical Manual II (DSM II R)*, revised edn, Washington, DC: American Psychiatric Press.

Ames G.M. (1989) 'Alcohol-Related Movements and their Effects on Drinking Policies in the American Workplace: An Historical Review,' *Journal of Drug Issues* Fall 19 (4): 489–510.

Anderson, D. (1989) 'The Current Debate About Alcohol: Extreme Allegations and Sobering Evidence', in D. Anderson (ed.), *Drinking to Your Health: The Allegations and the Evidence*, London: Social Affairs Unit.

Babor, T and Willetts, J. (1986) 'Alcohol-Related Problems in the Primary Health Care Setting : A Review of Early Intervention Studies', *British Journal of Addiction* 81: 23–47.

Belle-Glass, I. and Marshall, J. (1991) 'Alcohol and Mental Illness: Cause or Effect?', in I. Belle-Glass (ed.), *The International Book of Addiction Behaviour*, London: Routledge.

Bennett, D. (1994) *Health Gain Investment Programme: Technical Review Document*, Trent: NHS Executive, Trent Regional Health Authority.

Bennett, P. and Anthony, P. (1992) *Health Gain Investment Programme: Technical Review Document*, Trent: NHS Executive, Trent Regional Health Authority.

Bennett, P. and Hodgson, R. (1992) 'Psychology and Health Promotion', in R. Bunton and G. MacDonald (eds), *Health Promotion – Disciplines and Diversity*, London: Routledge.

Cadoret, R.J. and Gath, A. (1978) 'Inheritance of Alcoholism in Adoptees', *British Journal of Psychiatry* 132: 252–8.

Chick, J., Harris, B. and Evans, M. (1985) 'Counselling Problem Drinkers in Medical Wards', *British Medical Journal* March 30: 965–967.

Cooper, A.M. (1989) 'How Different Societies Learn to Drink: Well and Badly', in D. Anderson (ed.), *Drinking to Your Health: The Allegations and the Evidence*, London: Social Affairs Unit.

Delgado, M. (1990) 'Hispanic Adolescent and Substance Abuse: Implications for Research, Treatment and Prevention', in A.R. Stiffman and L.E. Davis (eds), *Ethnic Issues in Adolescent Mental Health*, London: Sage.

DOH (1989) *Alcohol Misuse*, Health Circular HN (89) 4, London: DOH.

—— (1992) *The Health of the Nation: A Strategy for Health in England*, London: HMSO.

Dillner, L. (1991) 'Alcohol Abuse – the Problem has not Gone Away', *British Medical Journal* April 13: 859–860.

Drummond, D.C. (1991) 'Dependence on Psychoactive Drugs: Finding a Common Language', in I. Belle-Glass (ed.), *The International Book of Addiction Behaviour*, London: Routledge

Edwards, E.D. and Egbert-Edwards, M. (1990) 'American–Indian Adolescent: Combating Problems of Substance Use and Abuse Through a Community Model', in A.R. Stiffman and L.E. Davis (eds), *Ethnic Issues in Adolescent Mental Health*, London: Sage.

Freeman, E. (1990) 'Social Competence as a Framework for Addressing Ethnicity and Teenage Alcohol Problems', in A.R. Stiffman and L.E. Davis (eds), *Ethnic Issues in Adolescent Mental Health*, London: Sage.

Garretson, H. and Goor, I. (1992) 'Harm Reduction and Alcohol', *International Journal on Drug Policy* 3 (4): 168–169.

General Household Survey (1992) London: Government Statistics Office.

—— (1995) London: Government Statistics Office.

Grant, M. and Ritson, B. (1983) *Alcohol – The Prevention Debate*, London: Croom Helm.

Grant, N. and Hodgson, R. (eds) (1991) *Responding to Drug and Alcohol Problems in the Community*, Geneva: WHO.

Green, L. and Raeburn, J. (1990) 'Contemporary Developments in Health Promotion Definitions and Challenges', in N. Bracht, *Health Promotion at the Community Level*, London: Sage.

Health Education Authority (1991) *HEA Response to Health of the Nation*, London: HEA.

—— (1993) *Health Update 3: Alcohol*, London: HEA.

Heath, D. (1989) 'Policies, Politics and Pseudoscience: A Cautionary Tale about Alcohol Controls', in D. Anderson (ed.), *Drinking to Your Health: The Allegations and the Evidence*, London: Social Affairs Unit.

Hutcheson, F. (1988) 'Growing Threats to Public Health', in A. Smith and B. Jacobson (eds), *The Nation's Health*, Oxford: Oxford University Press.

Jessor, R. and Jessor, S.L. (1975) 'Adolescent Development and the Onset of Drinking: A Longitudinal Study', *Journal of the Study of Alcohol* 36: 27–51.

—— (1977) *Problem Behaviour and Psychological Development: A Longitudinal Study of Growth*, New York: Academic Press.

Kaji, L. (1966) 'Alcoholism in Twins, Stockholm, Sweden', in A. Almqvist and D. Wiksell, *Studies on the Aetiology and Sequels of Abuse of Alcohol*, Lund: University of Lund, Department of Psychiatry.

Kandel, D. (1982) 'Epidemiological and Psychosocial Perspective on Adolescent Drug Use', *Journal of American Academic Clinical Psychiatry* 21: 238 –347.

Kendell. R., Walport, M. and Rynes, R. (1983) 'Influence of an Increase in Excise Duty on Consumption and its Adverse Effects', *British Medical Journal* September 17: 809–811.

Labouvie, E.W. (1986) 'Alcohol and Marijuana Use in Relation to Adolescent Stress', *International Journal of Addiction* 21: 33–345.

Levine, H.G. (1992) 'Temperature Cultures: Alcohol as a Problem of Nordic English Speaking Cultures', in M. Lader, G. Edwards and D.C. Drummond (eds), *The Nature of Alcohol and Drug-related Problems*, New York: Oxford University Press.

May, P.A. and Moran, J.R. (1995) 'Prevention of Alcohol Misuse: a Review of Health Promotion Effort among American Indians', *American Journal of Health Promotion* April 9, 4: 286–299.

Maynard, A. (1991) 'Economic Aspects of the Markets for Alcohol, Tobacco and Illicit Drugs', in I. Belle-Glass (eds), *The International Book of Addiction Behaviour*, London: Routledge.

Mulford, H.A. (1994) 'What if Alcoholism Had Not Been Invented? The Dynamics of American Alcohol Mythology', *Addiction* May, 89 (5): 517–524.

Nobles, E., Goddard, L.L., Cavil, W.E. and George, P.Y. (1987) *The Culture of Drugs in the Black Community*, Oakland, CA: Black Family Institute, pp.10–36.

O'Connor, J. (1978) *The Young Drinkers: A Cross-national Study of Social and Cultural Influences*, London: Tavistock.

Ogborne, A. and Smart, R. (1980) 'Will Restriction on Advertising Reduce Alcohol Consumption?', *British Journal of Addiction*, 75: 293–296.

Oyemade, U. (1985) 'Achievement of Black Adolescents in Academic and Non-academic Areas', in *Proceedings of Symposium: The Ecology of Black Adolescents. Symposium Conducted at the Meeting of the Society for Research in Child Development, Toronto, Canada*, Chicago IL: University of Chicago Press.

Oyemade, U. and Washington, V. (1990) 'The Role of Family Factors in the Primary Prevention of Substance Abuse among High-risk Black Youth', in A.R. Stiffman and L.E. Davis (eds), *Ethnic Issues in Adolescent Mental Health*, London: Sage.

Partanen, J., Bruun, K. and Markkanen, T. (1966) *Inheritance of Drinking Behaviour*, Helsinki: Finnish Foundation for Alcohol Studies, pp. 14–159.

Peele, S. (1993) 'The Conflict between Public Health Goal and the Temperance Mentality', *American Journal of Public Health* 83: 803–810.

—— (1996) 'Utilizing Culture and Behaviour in Epidemiological Models of Alcohol Consumption and Consequences for Western Nations', *Alcohol and Alcoholism* 32.

Peterson, M. and Johnstone, B.M. (1995) 'The Atwood Hall Health Promotion Program, Federal Medical Centre, Lexington, Kentucky: Effects on Drug-involved Federal Offenders', *Journal of Substance Abuse Treatment* January–February, 12 (1): 43–48.

Posner, N. (1992) *Plans Into Action: Three Case Studies of Regional Alcohol Studies*, London: The Tavistock Institute.

Roberts, R. (1988) 'Hiccups in Alcohol Education', *Health Education Journal* 47 (2 and 3): 73–76.

Rowland, P. and Maynard, B. (1993) 'Alcohol Education: Does it Work?', *Guardian*, 22 February: 4.

Royal College of Physicians (1991) *Community Medicine* 28 (3): 223–5, Bristol: Royal College of Physicians.

Royal College of Psychiatrists (1986) *Alcohol Our Favourite Drug*, London: Tavistock Publications.

Rutherford, D. (1993) 'WHO Targets Europe with Alcohol Action Plan', *Alcohol Alert* February: 1–3.

Saunders, P. (1992) 'Drinkwise', Portman Group Publications, pp. 1–4, London.

Saunders, W. (1984) 'Alcohol Use in Britain: How Much is too Much?' *Health Education Journal* 43 (2 and 3): 66–70.

—— (1987) 'Who Keeps the Alcohol Industry Afloat?', *Canadian School Health Journal* 10 (February): 131–135.

Schuckit, M.A. (1987) 'Studies of Populations at High risk for the Future Development of Alcoholism', H. W. Goedde and D.P. Agarwal (eds), *Genetics of Alcoholism*, New York: Alan Liss.

Stiffman, A.R. and Davis, L.E.(eds) (1990) *Ethnic Issues in Adolescent Mental Health*, London: Sage.

Tones, K. (1987) 'Devising Strategies for Preventing Drug Misuse: The Role of the Health Action Model', *Health Education Research* 2 (4): 305–317.

—— (1990) *Health Education Effectiveness and Efficiency*, London: Chapman & Hall.

Velleman, R. (1992) *Counselling for Alcohol Problems*, London: Sage.

Wallace, S. (1993) 'The Development of Alcohol Strategies in England and Wales', *Journal of the Royal Society of Medicine* 86, June: 319–323.

Wells, B. (1991) 'Self-help Groups', in I. Belle-Glass (eds), *The International Book of Addiction Behaviour*, London: Routledge.

West, R. (1991) 'Psychological Theories of Addiction', in I. Belle-Glass (eds), *The International Book of Addiction Behaviour*, London: Routledge.

WHO (1985) *Targets for Health for All*, Geneva: WHO.

—— (1986) 'Lifestyles and Health, Regional Office for Europe, Health Education Unit', *Social Science and Medicine* 22 (2): 117–124.

Williams, G. (1993) 'Britain's Flight from Alcohol: The Reality of Non-drinking in the 1990's', *Alcohol Alert* February Supplement: 2–15.

Zeitlin, H. and Swadi, H. (1991) 'Adolescence: the Genesis of Addiction', in I. Belle-Glass (ed.), *The International Book of Addiction Behaviour*, London: Routledge.

Chapter 14

Campbell, D. and Stanley, J. (1963) *Experimental and Quasi Experimental Designs for Research*, Chicago, IL: Rand McNally.

COMMIT (1995) 'Community Intervention Trial for Smoking Cessation: Cohort Results from a Four Year Intervention', *American Journal of Public Health* 85: 183–192.

Cook, T.D. (1985) 'Postpositivism Critical Multiplism', in L. Shortland and M.M. Mark (eds), *Social Science and Policy*, Newbury Park, CA : Sage, pp. 21–62.

Douglas, J., Ross, J. and Simpson, H. (1971) *All Our Future,* New York: Peter Davies, Panther.

Downie, R.S., Fyfe, C. and Tannahill, A. (1990) *Health Promotion: Models and Values*, Oxford: Oxford University Press.

Epp, J. (1986) *Achieving Health for All: A Framework for Health Promotion*, Ottawa: Health and Welfare, Canada.

Fetterman, D., Kaftarian, S. and Wandersman, A. (eds) (1996) *Empowerment Evaluation: Knowledge and Tools for Self-Assessment and Accountability*, London: Sage.

Goodstadt, M.S., Simpson, R.I. and Loranger, P.O. (1987) 'Health Promotion: A Conceptual Integration', *American Journal of Health Promotion* Winter: 58–63.

Green, L.W. (1980) 'Current Report: Office of Health Information, Health Promotion Physical Fitness and Sports Medicine', *Health Education* March/April: 28.

Green, L.W. and Kreuter, M.M. (1991) *Health Promotion Planning: An Educational and Environmental Approach*, Mountain View, CA: Mayfield.

Green, L.W. and Ottoson, J.M. (1994) *Community Health*, 7th edn, St Louis, MO: Mosby, p. 700.

Green, L.W. and Raeburn, J. (1990) 'Contemporary Developments in Health Promotion: Definitions and Challenges', in N. Bracht (ed.), *Health Promotion at the Community Level*, Newbury Park, CA: Sage.

Green, L. and Richard, L. (1993) 'The Need to Combine Health Education and Health Promotion: The Case of Cardiovascular Disease Prevention', *Promotion and Education* 1: 11–17.

REFERENCES

Hart, J. (1994) *Feasible Socialism – The NHS: Past, Present and Future*, London: Socialist Health Association, pp. 36–38.

Kickbusch, I. (1994) 'Introduction: Tell Me a Story', in A. Pederson, M. O'Neill and I. Rootman (eds), *Health Promotion in Canada: Provincial, National and International Perspectives*, Toronto: W.B. Saunders.

Labonte, R. and Little, S. (1992) *Determinants of Health: Empowering Strategies for Nurses*, Vancouver: Registered Nurses Association of British Columbia.

Lalonde, M. (1974) *A New Perspective on the Health of Canadians*, Ottawa: Information Canada.

Martin, C.J. and McQueen, D.V. (eds) (1989) *Readings for a New Public Health*, Edinburgh: Edinburgh University Press.

NCI Breast Cancer Screening Consortium (1990) 'Screening Mammography: A Missed Clinical Opportunity? National Health Interview Survey Studies', *Journal of the American Medical Association* 264: 54–58.

Nutbeam, D., Smith, C. and Catford, J. (1990) 'Evaluation in Health Education: A Review of Progress, Possibilities and Problems', *Journal of Epidemiology and Community Health* 44: 83–89.

O'Donnell, M.P. (1989) 'Definition of Health Promotion: Part III – Expanding the Definition', *American Journal of Health Promotion* 3 (3): 5.

Patton, M.Q. (1982) *Practical Evaluation*, Newbury Park, CA: Sage.

Pederson, A., O'Neill, M. and Rootman, I. (1994) *Health Promotion in Canada: Provincial, National and International Perspectives*, Toronto: W.B. Saunders.

Potvin, L., and Macdonald, M. (1995) 'Methodological Challenges for the Evaluation of Dissemination Phase Health Promotion Programs, unpublished manuscript.

Rokeach, M. (1983) 'A Value Approach to the Prevention and Reduction of Drug Abuse', in T.J. Glynn, C.G. Leukefeld and J.P. Ludford (eds), *Preventing Adolescent Drug Abuse: Intervention Strategies*, Rockville, MD: US Public Health Service, Department of Health and Human Services, pp. 172–194.

Rootman, I., and Raeburn, J. (1994) 'The Concept of Heath', in A. Pederson, M. O'Neill and I. Rootman (eds), *Health Promotion in Canada: Provincial, National and International Perspectives*, Toronto: W.B. Saunders.

Rossi, P.H. and Freeman, H.E. (1989) *Evaluation: A Systematic Approach*, 4th edn, Newbury Park, CA: Sage.

Scriven, M. (1973) 'Goal-free Evaluation', in R.E. House (ed.), *School Evaluation: The Politics and Process*, Berkeley, CA: McCutchan, pp. 319–328.

Shadish, W.R., Cook, T.D. and Leviton, L.C. (1991) *Foundations of Program Evaluation: Theories of Practice*, Newbury Park, CA: Sage.

Shea, S. and Basch, C. (1990) 'A Review of Five Major Community-based Cardiovascular Disease Prevention Programs. Part II: Intervention Strategies, Evaluation Methods and Results', *American Journal of Health Promotion* 4: 279–287.

Springett, J. and Dugdill, L. (1995) 'Workplace Health Promotion Programmes: Towards a Framework for Evaluation', *Health Education Journal* 55: 91–103.

Springett, J., Costongs, C. and Dugdill, L. (1995) 'Towards a Framework for Evaluation in Health Promotion: the Importance of the Process, *Journal of Contemporary Health* 2: 61–65.

REFERENCES

Stachechenko, S and Jenicek, M. (1990) 'Conceptual Differences Between Prevention and Health Promotion: Research Implications for Community Health Programs', *Canadian Journal of Public Health* 81 (January/February): 53–59.

Susser, M. (1975) 'Epidemiological Models', in E. Struening and M. Guttelag (eds), *Handbook of Evaluation Research*, Beverly Hills: Sage, pp. 497–517.

US Department of Health, Education and Welfare (1979) *Health People: The Surgeon General's Report of Health Promotion and Disease Prevention*, Washington, DC: Government Printing Office.

Wagner, E., Koespell, T. and Anderman, C. (1991) 'The Evaluation of the Henry J. Kaiser Family Foundation's Community Health Promotion Grant Program', *Journal of Clinical Epidemiology* 44: 685–699.

WHO (1984) *Discussion Document on the Concept and Principles of Health Promotion*, Copenhagen: European Office of the WHO.

—— (1987) 'Ottawa Charter for Health Promotion', *Health Promotion* 4: iii–v

INDEX